Praise for
Attention *Difference* Disorder®

*"Must Reading For All Parents
and ADHD Healthcare Professionals"*

"Dr. Kenny Handelman's approach to ADHD as a "difference" than as a "deficit" is a breakthrough concept, and one that every parent (and doctor) needs to learn and get on board with. These children have many strengths, and focusing on deficits is too often a self-fulfilling prophecy. Easy to read, and presenting just the basic facts of what parents need to know to progress from being ADHD students to becoming ADHD experts and advocates, is exactly the right approach.

Must reading for all parents and ADHD healthcare providers."

Dr. Peter Jensen

Co-Director, Division of Child Psychiatry & Psychology,

The Mayo Clinic, Rochester, MN

Author of: Making The System Work For Your Child With ADHD

"This Book Will Lead You From Frustration...
To Experiencing Success"

"Run, don't walk to the nearest book store and purchase your copy of *Attention Difference Disorder*, by Dr. Handelman. The understanding, practical strategies and hope you will gain from reading this book will lead you from frustration, dealing with ADD, to experiencing success and feelings of promise and possibility. Thank you Dr. Handelman for a much needed resource!!"

SHELLEY PETERS MERKEL, *Oakville, Canada*

"The First Chapter Alone Is Better
Than Anything Else We Have Ever Read"

"We have raised two children with ADD and the first chapter alone in Dr. Handelman's book is better than anything else we have ever read or studied. The Attention Difference Disorder 7 step system makes the overwhelming task of raising a child with ADD much more simple.

As experienced parents, we found this book tremendously helpful. If you are just starting out - this book is an indispensible resource.

If you and your child want to be successful, this is the best book you could read and study."

ALAN AND HOLLY REED, *Idaho Falls, ID*

"Thanks For Providing The Steps
Needed To Make A Difference"

"As a father, I wish I could've had this book 20 years ago! This book answered a lot of questions for me and gave me a lot of "ah ha's" as to things I didn't even relate to being associated to ADD and how to use those 'differences' as a positive. Thanks Dr. Kenny, for providing the steps needed to make a difference."

FRANK DEARDURFF, *Terre Haute, Indiana*

"*It Can Literally Be a Lifesaver!*"

"When I found out that my daughter was diagnosed with ADD, I can honestly say that I was confused and puzzled for days. I clearly had a "what now?" look on my face. I spent days researching ADD/ADHD, and tried to figure out on my own what would help our daughter, and what was simply a myth. We were finally able to turn her deficiencies into strengths, but a lot of it was trial and error.

Had I know about Dr. Handelman's book, it could have saved us weeks—maybe months—of stress, fear and uncertainty. The information presented within is clear, and the steps are actionable. Most important, it's written at a level that any parent can understand, without having to figure out unclear medical jargon. I now use the book as a "refresher course", to consistently maintain a level of stability in our daughter's development, and the result has been nothing short of amazing. I highly recommend the book to parents of ADD/ADHD children, and anyone wishing to get a better grasp of the condition—it can literally be a lifesaver!"

"DJ" DAVE BERNSTEIN, *Phoenix, Arizona* www.HiFiWebGuy.com

"*This Book Can Absolutely Turn Your Child's Struggles Upside Down*"

"Attention Difference Disorder might strike you as odd or going against the curve, but Dr. Handelman not only shows you why this new perspective makes sense, but he backs up with concrete science and clinical experience. This book, but more importantly, this perspective is one that can absolutely turn your child's struggles upside down and give you the loving, confident, successful child you have been asking yourself if it is truly possible. With this book, and Dr. Handelman as your guide, it absolutely is."

RORY F. STERN, PSYD, *www.ADHDFamilyOnline.com*

"I Knew This Was The Book I've Been Looking For"

"ATTENTION DIFFERENCE DISORDER is an amazing book.

I feel like it was written for me rather than someone that's seeking to obtain a medical degree in the area of ADD. Shortly after I picked it up I knew this was the book that I've been looking for. As a parent, I found the chapters on the "Parent's ADD Journey" and Parenting Strategies extremely helpful. Thanks again; my wife will be reading this next."

TRACY C., *Father in Cordova, TN*

"You Include Extensive Parenting Strategies"

"I wanted to start by saying this book is great! It is the all encompassing, well written, and easy to understand book that every parent can use as they begin their ADHD journey with their child. It was so much easier to read your book than the resources that were available to me when my son was first diagnosed. I appreciate how you take a look at all the options that are available to parents and children. Many books don't take the time to include such extensive parenting strategies the way you do. This is such a key factor for long term success. I got some great tips and reminders of things I need to work on."

SEANA CAMPBELL-WOOD, *Oakville, Canada*

"So Easy To Read"

"After reading "Attention Difference Disorder" I breathed a huge sigh of relief. I finally found the answers to so many frustrating problems my family had been living with for years. We all finally understand why we act and feel the way we do. We're not freaks, just different. Now we have practical tactics that have made a dramatic difference in life at home and at school. It was so easy to read, not full of unintelligible technical jargon. Even for my child who doesn't have ADHD, I learned some very good parenting techniques that help avoid the feeling, "I wish this kid came with an instruction book!" Thank you Dr. Handelman. You've made a big difference."

JULIE VERRINDER, *Salt Lake City, Utah*

"Learn to Embrace Your Difference, Not Fight Against it."

"As an adult who has ADD and is also a parent of a young adult child with ADHD, I am thrilled to see that someone finally has the guts to take a stand for the people who are blessed with this "difference." I always taught my son that ADD could be his biggest asset, as it is mine, if he learned how to channel it properly. Dr. Handelman is teaching people what I had to struggle through to discover on my own; to embrace their difference, not fight against it. This concise and easy to understand book is long overdue. Thank you Dr. Handelman!"

VICKI CONLEY, *Lake Lanier, Georgia*

KENNY HANDELMAN, M.D.

Attention
Difference
Disorder®

How to Turn Your
ADHD Child or Teen's
Differences into Strengths
in **7 SIMPLE STEPS**

MORGAN JAMES PUBLISHING • NEW YORK

Attention *Difference* Disorder

ISBN: 978-1-60037-846-1 (Paperback)
Library of Congress Control Number: 2010933818

Published by:
MORGAN JAMES PUBLISHING
1225 Franklin Ave Ste 32, Garden City, NY 11530-1693
Toll Free 800-485-4943   www.MorganJamesPublishing.com

Cover/Interior Design by:
Rachel Lopez
rachel@r2cdesign.com

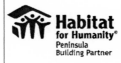

Dedication

This book, *Attention Difference Disorder*, is dedicated to Cheryl and Keleila. Thank you for all of your love and support.

Table of Contents

Acknowledgements

I didn't enter medical school wanting to specialize in ADHD. Ending up as an expert in ADHD was a gradual process, influenced as it was by my teachers, supervisors and mentors. I was lucky to have great supervisors and educators who both taught and inspired me. For example, I appreciate the important role played by Dr. Marshall Korenblum who helped to spark my interest in child and adolescent psychiatry. And my thanks to Dr. Russell Schachar and Dr. Abel Ickowicz, both of whom gave me great training and experience with ADHD when I was at Toronto's Hospital for Sick Children. They taught me well, and sparked an intense professional interest which has ultimately led to this book—an interest which will continue to grow as I continue my work in ADHD.

Once professionally engaged in the field of ADHD, I have had many colleagues who have taught and inspired me. I want to acknowledge Dr. Russell Barkley. Dr. Barkley is one of the top researchers in ADHD, and I have learned so much from his research, presentations and his books. Listening to him present is an absolute treat—he packs so much information and up-to-date research into his presentations. Thank you for teaching me so much about the field.

Another major influence for me is Dr. Edward Hallowell. Dr. Hallowell has been an author, speaker and strong advocate for ADHD for many years. I remember reading his *Driven to Distraction* when I was in my residency and just starting to learn about ADHD. I subsequently had the privilege of meeting and then presenting with him. On studying the body of his work I have been made aware of and gained great appreciation for the contribution that he has made to this field and to my thinking and understanding of ADHD. He has helped to shape my strength-based view of ADHD. And I am grateful that he agreed to write the foreword for this book. Thanks Ned!

Writing a book is a bigger task than I ever imagined. I want to thank the team at Morgan James: to David Hancock for his support for this book right from the time it was just an idea, and to Jim Howard, and Margo Toulouse. I also want to thank John Maling—Editor in Chief of Mile High Press and The Book Shepherd. Thank you for your editing efforts. I have to say that you provided me the best surprise about writing my first book—you took my words, and made me sound clearer and better. Thank you so much for that!

I could not do what I do without the love and support of my family. I am privileged to have wonderful parents, Arny and Elaine, and three outstanding siblings: Jill, Judi and David. Then we've added John, Martine, Simone and Tamara (and a new niece or nephew, due before this book hits print!). I appreciate the love and support that you have all showed me over the course of my life. And special thanks and appreciation go to Cheryl and Keleila. I love you both so much, and I appreciate how much support you've shown me—as I was out presenting on ADHD, or had my home office door closed, writing or working until the late hours.

I feel that it is critically important to acknowledge the brave kids, teens and adults that I've had the privilege of working with over more than a decade of my professional involvement with ADHD. I have learned so much from the journeys that you have taken, and shared with me. I am honored that I have been able to contribute to your lives, and to help you to achieve what you are capable of. There are so many patients who have overcome what they were told they shouldn't be able to—patients who have inspired me tremendously. I can say without hesitation that my patients have taught me more about what is possible with ADHD than any other source of understanding. It is my patients' successes (through their hard work) which have played a big role in inspiring me and changing my perspective to see the potential positives and opportunities within ADHD.

Finally, I acknowledge you—the reader. Clearly, this book has entered into your hands, and if you are this far into the acknowledgments, then no doubt you are on a journey with ADD/ADHD. Thank you for your interest in *Attention Difference Disorder*.

My advice?

Read on, there are answers and support for you in the pages ahead...

Foreword

I first met Canadian psychiatrist Kenny Handelman in 2007 at a seminar in Scottsdale, Arizona. I was immediately struck by his warmth, energy and enthusiasm as well as his fervent desire to educate the general public on issues related to mental health, particularly those pertaining to attention deficit hyperactivity disorder, or ADHD.

As a psychiatrist and author myself, I share Kenny's passion for sharing what we doctors know. Nowhere in all of medicine does the public's use of what the science knows lag further behind than it does in mental health. We desperately need qualified practitioners who can translate the science into words the public can understand, appreciate, and use to relieve suffering and promote health, happiness, and productivity. We dearly need to eliminate the stigma and ignorance that have so plagued the field of mental health for centuries, as we pay a huge price, both emotionally as well as financially due its devastating effects.

To that end, it is with great pleasure and gratitude that I greet this new book by Dr. Handelman and offer these few words of introduction.

Kenny—let me call him Kenny, as that is how I know him—works in the trenches treating ADHD in children and adults. He is a practitioner first and foremost, which makes him all the more trustworthy. Not only does he have the credentials to back up what he writes, he also has the direct and invaluable experience with patients.

He's been percolating this book for quite a while. That he has given it much thought is apparent because the book is so clear. Writers who don't really know their subject tend to write confusing books. Writers who know their subject well, write with clarity and punch.

Not only is Kenny's writing clear and vivid, his advice is practical and easy to use. He doesn't require the reader to work hard; he's already done the work.

His elegant organizational scheme—the seven steps—corrals the essentials on ADHD and offers them up in easy-to-digest chapters. The reader will almost feel as if Kenny were right there in the room, explaining and pausing, then moving on to the next subject. While he won't be able to stop and ask, "Any questions?" you might feel as if he could.

This is a book a person who knows nothing about ADHD can read, but it is also a book someone who already knows a lot can benefit from reading as well. One of the many charms of the book is the ease with which it shifts from elementary to advanced level without losing a step.

If you are looking for an authoritative but also accessible and hopeful guide to the world of ADHD, this is the book for you. You will learn about diagnosis and you will learn about treatment. You will learn about medication and you will learn about treatments that do not involve medication. You will learn about the orthodox, scientifically validated treatments, and you will learn about some of the alternative treatments that hold promise. As we await research into these new treatments, it is useful to know which ones appear most likely to become mainstream and which do not.

As a doctor who has been treating ADHD in children and adults for 30 years, and as an author who's written six books on various aspects of ADHD, I can state with certainty that ADHD can cripple a child or an adult. I can also state with certainty that proper diagnosis and treatment can not only free the individual from the chaos and pain ADHD can create, but also propel that individual to magnificent success.

One of my most fervent missions in life is to bring the good news about diagnosis and treatment of ADHD to the tens of millions of people who still live in the darkness created by stigma and ignorance. Untreated, ADHD can create a dark world indeed, leading to academic failure, depression, anxiety, substance abuse, violent behavior, accidents, trauma, rampant underachievement, inability to sustain relationships or keep jobs in adulthood, and even incarceration or suicide. Untreated, ADHD can ruin the life of an individual as well as a family.

But, this is a preventable tragedy. With the knowledge we have at our fingertips, knowledge Dr. Handelman so skillfully and clearly lays out in this fine book, any parent, teacher, friend, or spouse—any interested individual— can see to it that the person who has ADHD gets the help that can not only prevent the damage but promote the successes that people with ADHD are capable of achieving.

People with ADHD have won Nobel Prizes and Pulitzer Prizes. People with ADHD have become billionaire entrepreneurs. People with ADHD have become brain surgeons, trial attorneys, movie stars, professional athletes, CEO's, Generals, Admirals, and leaders of all kinds in all professions. As deeply as untreated ADHD can scar a person, treatment can open the door for that person to achieve extraordinary success and happiness.

That's the good news. And what good news it is. The knowledge in this book can change lives *dramatically* for the better. The knowledge in this book can put an end to years of suffering. The knowledge in this book can turn lives completely around.

All you, the reader, need do is read on. Then take action. Consult with a professional who has experience in treating ADHD. It is critical you see someone who has experience, as many practitioners don't know what they don't know, and so cannot give you the best help.

But, armed with the knowledge in this book, and the help of an experienced professional, you can turn the life of your child who has ADHD around, or the life of your spouse, or your own life.

Thanks to Dr. Handelman's clear and reliable guide, you're ready to go. You're ready to lay claim to the life you—or your loved one—ought to have. Now, let knowledge do its work. Let knowledge shine the light and put an end to the darkness and the pain.

Good luck!

—Edward Hallowell, M.D.

Introduction

there is a vast amount of information available to you right now. Depending on how you access the internet, you can probably turn on your smart phone and tap into the biggest database of information that has ever existed—the internet—right in the palm of your hand. And while there is so much information available to you, it can also be overwhelming. It can be hard to know which resources to trust, and it can be hard to sift through the massive volumes of information which are available in order to find what is relevant to you.

This book is the distillation of my 10+ years of working with ADD/ADHD, as well as attending conferences, reading research, and presenting the information I have gleaned, to people just like yourself. As a board certified Psychiatrist in the USA and Canada, and an expert in ADD and ADHD, I often teach medical students, doctors, parents, educators and others about ADD/ADHD.

Presenting ADD/ADHD, as I have, to so many different audiences has helped me to sift through that immense amount of information to present what is relevant just to you. I have heard and responded to many, many different questions asked, and I have incorporated the answers to those wide-ranging questions into the information that you'll read in this book. My mission is to make sure that my reader (you) get the right information you need, at the time you need it, to make the best healthcare decisions you can. This book will help you to do just that.

One of the biggest challenges with ADD is that there are so many myths and misconceptions out there among the uninformed. People become confused, may not accept the diagnosis of ADD/ADHD and, as a result, refuse treatments that help. As a parent, you always want to be sure that you are making the best decisions for your child. When you hear conflicting messages about ADD or the treatments for ADD, making a choice can be very difficult out of fear that you may be harming your child.

The goal of this book is to give you the *right* information, right now. It is intended to correct the misconceptions, eliminate any confusion, and help you to make informed choices about ADD/ADHD for your child or teen.

As an expert in ADD/ADHD, my goal is to condense the vast amount I've learned in the field during my professional career into a relatively small number of easy-to-read pages. I intend to use my more than 10 years of experience seeing kids, teens and adults with ADD/ADHD, to share practical and useful tips that will make this journey easier for you.

> First things first — for the purposes of this book the acronym "ADD" will refer to both ADD and ADHD. Please know that this term is intended to cover all aspects of the condition—whether hyperactivity is involved in the condition or not.

The Goals of This Book

The four goals of this book are:

1) To break down misconceptions/myths.

2) To get you to think differently about ADD.

3) To have you realize that there are *differences* within ADD rather than *deficits*.

4) To be easy to read.

Goal #1: To Break Down Misconceptions & Myths

The case with ADD is when the misconceptions are eliminated, and treatment begins (whatever that treatment may be) there can be dramatic improvements. That includes improvements with the core symptoms of ADD—such as inattention, hyperactivity and impulsivity.

Additionally, the improvements can go far beyond just the core symptoms. When ADD is treated, improvements can include:

- Improved self esteem,
- Better social functioning,
- Improved academic and occupational functioning,
- Better relationships,
- And a whole lot more …

On the flip side, the consequences of not treating ADD can be problematic—significantly so. Numerous studies clearly show that people with untreated ADD are at risk of significant long term consequences—consequences such as:

- Academic underachievement,
- Poor work functioning,
- Increased risk of drug and alcohol use and addiction,
- Increased accidents and injuries,
- Poor social skills and trouble with friendships,
- Driving problems,
- And much more …

With erroneous information gone, it is much easier for real progress to be made with ADD. When you have the right information, it will be easier for you to eliminate any confusion and feel confident with the healthcare choices you are making for your children.

Goal #2: To Get You to Think Differently About ADD

As we clear away the misconceptions about ADD, we'll add the facts —with the most up-to-date science that's available.

Additionally, we'll move away from the purely negative, "disorder based" thinking of the standard medical approach. The standard medical approach to the concept of "disorder" serves people with ADD in many ways, but it can have its limitations as well.

For decades (possibly even centuries), people with ADD have been told to try harder and to stop "messing up." When ADD has been recognized as a real medical condition, it has helped the field tremendously. Medical science has begun to research the causes of ADD as well as the treatments. Funding has been developed for school programs, therapy programs, etc., and this was all achieved by the "medical approach" to ADD.

That said, I always feel uncomfortable telling little boys or girls that they are "disordered" because of the way they think. And the more I have gotten to know people with ADD, the more I have become aware of the fact that they are often incredible thinkers—creative, out of the box and original. Is that disordered? Well, it can be. But...

When the diagnostic criteria for ADD are met, we know that this is a disorder with long-term consequences. If we can get the disordered symptoms out of the way (through helpful, proven treatments), then we can allow the natural creativity to shine through, and ADD traits can become a strength.

This is one of the main differences I'd like you to think about with ADD. The fact that we can find and support strengths, and this can improve functioning, long term outcomes and—most importantly—self esteem.

Goal #3: There Are Differences with ADD Rather Than Deficits

ADD has been called many things over the years. The early terms included: Minimal Brain Damage, Minimal Brain Dysfunction, Hyperkinetic Disorder and others...

In 1980, the term "Attention Deficit" was introduced for this disorder.

The name "Attention Deficit" was quite helpful for the field. It helped people to focus on the inattention components of the condition, and move away from a purely "hyperactivity" view of the disorder (which would fail to include people who have ADD *without* hyperactivity). However, by using the term "deficit," it suggests that people with ADD have a complete deficit when it comes to attention, which, in fact, is not the case.

One of the first objections I get from parents of kids and teens who are first diagnosed is: "How can you say he has an attention *deficit*, when he can sit and play his video games for 12 hours if I didn't stop him? That's not much of a deficit."

After years of experience, it's my opinion that there is more of *difference* with attention rather than a *deficit*. Hence, the title of this book: *Attention Difference Disorder*. In Chapter 1, we'll cover the differences in more depth.

Goal #4: To Be a Book That Is Easy To Read

As a doctor on the "front lines" of assessment and treatment, it is my experience that there is usually one parent (often the mother, though not always) who generally comes to the appointments, and reads several books. Commonly, the second parent (often the dad) gets a cursory summary of ADD from the first parent, and often doesn't have time to get through a 300 page book on the subject. That is why this book intends to cover the important information that you need to know, with some different perspectives to help you, and in an easy-to-read format.

This book will not be 300 pages of technically worded, complicated science. I need to boil it down to the most important—the essential— information that you need. My goal is for this book to become an indispensible resource for you, your family and your treatment team.

I want this book to be so easy for you to read that you'll get through it, and in the process, become an expert in ADD. That will allow you to change your ADD child's life for the better.

What to Expect

In Chapter 1, I'll introduce the concept of Attention Difference Disorder, and share my rationale for using this term. I will introduce you to the Attention Difference Disorder System, which will help you to be thorough and complete in getting the help you need for your ADD child or teen.

Then, we'll talk about the "Parent's ADD Journey." This will help you to understand the nature of the challenge you have ahead of you, and the best way to view it.

What follows is one chapter for each of the "steps" in the Attention Difference Disorder System designed to help you to succeed in dealing with ADD.

The Seven Simple Steps to Succeed with ADD Are:

1) Step 1: Education about ADD
2) Step 2: Ensuring a proper assessment
3) Step 3: Parenting Strategies
4) Step 4: School and Academic Strategies
5) Step 5: Medication Treatment for ADD
6) Step 6: Alternative Treatments for ADD
7) Step 7: Treatment Integration

We'll then ask an important question: Can ADD be a gift? The answer will be addressed in one of our final chapters. Then, we'll wrap up with discussions on next steps and strategies for you.

Are the seven steps really simple?

The answer is yes and no.

Yes, the steps are simple because anyone can do them. All you need to do is to read this book, and then try the strategies in your own life. That is not hard. You do not need a PhD, or a medical degree to implement these steps.

And no, the steps aren't always simple; they depend on what your situation is and what your challenges are like. If you find that the steps aren't simple—it is not because the steps are hard, it is because of the challenges you are dealing with. If this is the case, then do your best to seek expert help (i.e. from a doctor, or therapist) in implementing the necessary steps. You will definitely need expert help working through the process of treating ADD in your child or teen.

Please note: this book is intended to support parents, caregivers and anyone who is working with ADD in kids and teens. *It is NOT intended to be a book on adult ADD.* Adult ADD creates a different set of challenges which will not be addressed here.

As mentioned, this book summarizes a lot of science for you. However, I have not included scientific references for most sections of this book; it is my job to summarize them for you. I have included scientific references for one chapter though—the chapter on alternative treatments for ADD. This was done in case you want to (or need to) share the scientific reference with your doctor or therapist when you begin a discussion about trying an alternative therapy with your child. While your doctor will agree with the science in all of the other chapters in this book, he or she may not agree with the proposed alternatives. Therefore, I have included the references so that you can help them to understand the research behind any particular treatment you'd like to undertake.

Let's get started…

CHAPTER 1

What's The Difference?

t his book begins with a bold title. Instead of calling the condition "Attention Deficit Disorder" (or "Attention Deficit Hyperactivity Disorder"), it is given a new name: "*Attention Difference Disorder.*"

History has changed the name of this condition several times, and let me be clear at the outset: it is not my intention to lobby to change the name officially to "Attention Difference Disorder." Rather, I want to help you to think *differently* about this condition. Words can be very powerful, and the difference between considering an attention *deficit* vs. an attention *difference* can be dramatic.

Is There Actually A Deficit In Attention?

ADD is diagnosed using criteria which are published by the American Psychiatric Association in the Diagnostic and Statistical Manual, 4th Edition, Text Revision (DSM-IV-TR). These criteria and how ADD is diagnosed will be covered in greater depth in Chapter 4. These criteria contain nine symptoms of inattention. These include: making careless mistakes, getting easily distracted, often being forgetful, and poor organization.

Based on the actual diagnostic criteria, there can be a deficit in attention. To even *be* diagnosed, one has to demonstrate quantitatively enough of the criteria which characterize these problems.

However, a diagnostic interview with parents and kids/teens can often go like this:

Doctor: "Does John have trouble paying close attention to details?"

Mom: "It depends…"

John: "Yeah… when I'm drawing, I can pay attention to the littlest details…"

Doctor: "Well, how about during math class?"

Mom: "Oh, well in math, there is a lot of trouble with that. But doesn't everyone find it harder to focus in math class?"

The point is this: when it comes to something you like, it's easier to pay attention to it. When it comes to something that you don't like, it's harder to pay attention to it. And while that can apply to everyone, the difference is dramatic in individuals with ADD.

When a doctor inquires about an inability to pay attention as part of the assessment for ADD, often he or she will ask about the areas that don't come as naturally and easily to the person, and also whether it occurs in a harder, more trying environment. For example, in a math class, while there are 25 other students in the room. The number of students is relevant, because if it is math class with a tutor providing one-to-one help, then it is easier for the child with ADD to focus.

Another way that a difference can manifest itself is when there is increased motivation for a particular topic. Even if your child with ADD struggles with a particular subject—let's say in a French class—and always has trouble with it, he or she can improve his or her focus if there is good reason to do so. For example, if Dad says: "John, if you pass your next French test, we'll get you the newest video game system as a reward." John will be incredibly motivated to succeed with his next test—especially if he has wanted that system for a long time. What would happen would be a disproportionate effort from John to succeed in his next French test, and he could actually do well with it. However, if he normally did well in his English class after French, he may not do well that day—because he's used up his attentional abilities on French.

Attention can vary by setting:

SETTINGS WITH MORE ATTENTION:	SETTINGS WITH LESS ATTENTION:
One on one work	Large groups
Fun and new	Boring and routine
Frequent feedback	Infrequent feedback
Supervised	Unsupervised
Fathers	Mothers
Strangers	Family
Clinic exam room	Waiting room

TABLE 1: Attention can vary by setting

In summary, it comes down to this: **There is a difference in attentional abilities in ADD.**

Is it always a deficit? Not necessarily.

But it is always a difference.

Now the critics of the condition will say: "ADD is not a real disorder—I mean, kids can focus on video games but not school work—that's just a fake disorder."

When helping to de-stigmatize mental health, I always like to bring forward other medical examples. The question becomes—are there other medical conditions which are symptomatic only under some circumstances yet not symptomatic in others?

Two examples are heart disease and asthma.

If you take your average adult male with heart disease, he doesn't have chest pains when he's sitting down and watching CSI reruns on TV. However, if he had to run up two flights of stairs, he would experience acute chest pain. In fact, the doctor could actually order a "stress test," i.e. the test will put him on a treadmill and make him run—a situation specifically designed to generate his chest pains!

Translation: In heart disease, people can have symptoms in some contexts, and lack symptoms in others.

For asthma, there are many people who get asthma attacks triggered by different things: cold weather, humidity, cat fur, allergies, etc. Again—their symptoms could be fine in one context, and then triggered in another.

So, even though people often criticize ADD as not being a true medical condition because there is no blood test or x-ray for it, shouldn't we allow ADD to have characteristics similar to other medical conditions like heart disease and asthma?

The point is clear: There is predominantly a difference in attention, which can manifest itself differently in different contexts.

Having established that kids and teens with ADD can focus better on areas that they like, we need to address a misconception often perpetuated by experts in the field. Doctors will often say that kids with ADD do better at subjects where they have to use their hands. They suggest that you should encourage your ADD child to go into the trades. While that may be great for some kids with ADD, I have seen many kids over the years with different strengths and passions. I've seen kids with ADD who read books for hours at home in their room (a quiet environment), or who love math class, or are great at computer programming. The message is simple—your ADD child may have talents in any academic area or interest—whether it is a thinking subject (reading, writing, math), or a doing subject (tech, or the trades).

The Implications of a Deficit

In 1968, Robert Rosenthal and Lenore Jacobson published results from a study called "Pygmalion in the Classroom." This study demonstrated that teacher expectations influenced students' achievement. What the researchers did was inform teachers that certain students' results on a written test showed that they had remarkable potential for academic growth. In fact, these students were chosen at random. When the researchers evaluated the progress of all students eight months later, the students whose teachers believed that they had great potential had the largest improvements in academic functioning.

While this study was done a long time ago, the message is clear. Most people live up to the expectations that people have of them. This is especially true for children and teens. And it's my personal belief that kids and teens live up to the negative expectations just as readily and easily as the positive expectations.

This is where we need to come back to the concept introduced in the introduction of this book. That by continually viewing ADD from a "disorder" perspective, we are setting up potential negative impacts. By telling boys and girls that they have deficits—we are setting up negative expectations for them and for what they may achieve in the future. My contention is that if we focus on "differences," we can still address the real medical issues involved with the disorder of ADD, yet not "pigeonhole" kids into a diagnosis and a label that can be detrimental.

Is this just "touchy feely," or "hokey," or some "new age" approach to walking on eggshells and being politically correct with wording?

My contention is a solid "No."

As a doctor in the field, it is my experience that the biggest negative consequence of ADD in the long run is shame.

When kids or teens have heard so many negative things about themselves, they can start to believe the "bad press." After so many times of trying hard, only to have parents or teachers say "Why don't you just apply yourself? You have so much potential…" After working hard to get friends only to find that an impulsive comment makes them leave for other people… After feeling that they know that they're smarter than kids getting A's or B's, but they just can't produce the work to get the marks…

Low self esteem develops, and shame and guilt set in.

And if the young person has the "good fortune" to go see a psychiatrist, psychologist or paediatrician (and "good fortune" is in quotes because, in my experience, most young people with ADD don't consider it good fortune to see a "head shrinker"), they are told that they have deficits and they are disordered.

This can be helpful in some ways however. Just having an explanation can help many people. That said, many kids and teens resist being labelled as disordered, and don't want to be considered different than other people.

This is where little differences can make a BIG difference. When a doctor is actually interested in what the child is good at, this is where it begins to matter. This is where, when the doctor seems to actually care, it matters to the teen. This is where focusing on strengths and opportunities can literally change a child or teen's perspective on participating in treatment and getting help … or resisting it with all of his or her might.

And talking about differences rather than deficits can make a BIG difference in the perception of the person that it counts most for: the child or teen whose self-esteem is suffering. It is this individual who needs to accept this diagnosis and treatment plan for things to really get better.

Deficits to Differences to Strengths

By following the steps in the Attention Difference Disorder System, you are going to learn to take the deficits that your child may have as part of their ADD and change them into differences. And as you move forward, you can convert those into strengths.

Repeating: One of the themes of this book is to take your child's deficits and turn them into differences, and then turn those differences into strengths.

Deficit → Difference → Strength

Taking Fire for This

Taking this stance on ADD has put me in the line of fire before, and I'm sure it will again.

Why?

Because there are doctors, researchers, experts, and people with ADD who suggest that looking at the strengths of ADD is irresponsible.

"We've worked long and hard to get the recognition for ADD as a real medical condition. Don't ruin it with this approach," they say.

Adults with ADD can say, "How can you consider the strengths in ADD, when my life has gone down the toilet because of this awful condition...?"

Some may challenge my character, or question my knowledge. And many will say: "Show me the science to prove that ADD has strengths in it. There isn't any..."

And I will listen to these criticisms, and the occasional personal attacks. And I will continue to have the same message:

There are differences, not deficits, and if we can get the disordered symptoms out of the way, and build on strengths, great things can come.

Having had the good fortune of helping many young people with ADD to succeed—and to find the strengths in their differences—I know that this approach can work. And I also know that it's worth carrying this message forward, even if it will cause occasional attacks on my credibility.

One child or teen's "thank you" for the help of getting their life on track—when they felt that previous approaches didn't help—is enough to propel me through hundreds if not thousands of attacks from people who don't see ADD this way.

In this book, I will share the science which has been shown to help ADD, and I will include my own approach and perspective which I have proven can be very helpful. My approach involves small differences; I find that sometimes small differences can make a big difference over time.

What about Hyperactivity?

We've spent time talking mainly about "attention differences" and we haven't yet spoken about hyperactivity. When researchers look at the prevalence of ADD, they find that the hyperactive-impulsive subtype is the least frequent manifestation of ADD in kids and teens. It is often reported as less than 10 percent. When it comes to the most common presentations, it is the combined subtype (i.e. having both the inattention and the hyperactive-impulsive subtype) followed by the inattentive subtype of ADD.

The bottom line here is that all of the strategies discussed in this book will work whether your main concern is inattentive ADD, hyperactive- impulsive ADD or combined ADD. We'll explore the subtypes of ADD in more detail in Chapter 3.

The Other Differences with ADD

There are other important differences in individuals with ADD as well. There are brain differences, genetic differences, as well as the ability to *hyperfocus*.

Brain research has progressed dramatically in the past 20 years. In the past, it was very hard to image the brain and reliably see what was going on while someone was alive and still using their brain. Now that technology has improved significantly; researchers are now doing brain imaging research regularly and they are dramatically increasing the science behind ADD. The brain research says the following:

There are brain differences in people with ADD.

This helps the credibility of the diagnosis of ADD, and is very important. And it is important to note that some of the treatment studies show that with good treatment for ADD, the brain differences resolve.

Family studies have shown that ADD is heritable—meaning that it runs in families. And researchers are actively looking for the genes which are involved in ADD. There are several "candidate genes" which have been identified, and research is ongoing.

One final "difference" to mention is the ability to *hyperfocus*. This difference presents an interesting paradox. People with ADD, who have trouble focusing attention, can increase that ability and actually focus more intently than normal—by hyperfocusing. The word hyperfocus means that there is an increase in the ability to focus on one area, often to the exclusion of other areas. People with ADD may be completely distractible, but in a crisis, they ignore everything else and hyperfocus on the issue at hand. An example: high school students who wait until the deadline approaches and then hyperfocus to get an assignment done. Hyperfocusing is another difference in ADD which can be used to people's advantage. You can harness the hyperfocusing ability by setting deadlines and using timers to induce the pressure often needed for ADD kids and teens to get things done.

CHAPTER 2

The "Parent's ADD Journey"

before beginning to review the steps in the Attention Difference Disorder System necessary to succeed with ADD, it's important for parents to be aware of a common "journey" which happens with many parents of ADD kids and teens.

I call it the "Parent's ADD Journey."

Why do parents end up knowingly or unknowingly taking this "journey"?

Because they have to...

The reality is that in many communities, it's hard for families to find experts in ADD who are able to assess and treat their kids in the short term, or provide monitoring for the long term. That's why it's so important for parents to become experts in ADD. In many cases, parents have to educate their own doctors about this condition.

This has always seemed absurd to me—patients having to teach their own doctors... I couldn't imagine it in the area of cardiology or respirology, where doctors (even primary care family doctors) are experts. However, when it comes to mental health, particularly ADD, most doctors didn't learn enough about it in medical school, and they certainly aren't up to date. Therefore, knowing more about ADD helps your child or teen's medical care and becomes very important for achieving satisfactory outcomes. Of course there are outstanding medical experts in ADD in many communities, and you may be lucky enough to have one as your doctor.

And in many schools, the educators have some understanding about ADD—but often not enough. There are certainly outstanding schools and educators out there, and they deserve all of the credit that they are due. That said, there are still many families who struggle because the school doesn't provide the support that their child needs; and they feel that they need to advocate and educate to get the help that their child needs and deserves.

What is the "Parent's ADD Journey"?

It can be summarized here:

Student ➜ Expert ➜ Advocate

Step 1: Becoming a Student of ADD:

Parents begin their "ADD Parent's Journey" as a *student* of the condition. They have many questions—about the diagnosis, the treatment, the strategies for home and school, There's a lot to learn about this condition to succeed with it.

ADD is not a condition for which you just take one pill in the morning and everything is OK. There's a lot more to it. And that's why education for ADD is Step 1 in the 7-Step, Attention Difference Disorder System.

And it doesn't matter how much one knows about ADD—one always needs to be a student of it. This is the reason that I attend several conferences and meetings each year to keep up to date on the newest developments with this condition.

Step 2: Becoming an Expert in ADD:

The next step in the "ADD Parent's Journey" is becoming an *expert*. The definition of expert at the website *www.Dictionary.com* is: "a person who has special skill or knowledge in some particular field; specialist; authority."

In my experience, becoming an expert is relative. In other words, it depends on who you are talking to—and whether they know more or less than you do. Many parents do not feel like an expert when they are seeing the specialist in ADD. However, they ARE an expert when they are talking to the teacher at school, the soccer coach, family members or even, sometimes, the family doctor.

Once parents learn specific facts and information about ADD, they are an expert compared to many people.

Even more importantly, they are THE expert on how ADD manifests with their child, and which strategies can work best with their child (once these have been understood with the help of the treating professionals).

And it is critically important for parents to give themselves credit for being the expert that they are, because of the next step that is needed in the "ADD Parent's Journey"...

Step 3: Becoming an Advocate for ADD:

This is the natural next step which parents need to progress to.

The definition of *advocate* on *www.dictionary.com* is:

NOUN: "a person who speaks or writes in support or defence of a person, cause, etc."

VERB: "to speak or write in favor of; support or urge by argument; recommend publicly."

Of course, one can "be an advocate for ADD"—i.e. this is a noun. And one can "advocate for the rights of people with ADD"—in this case it is a verb.

Sometimes, parents find that their kids are getting the right help—the help that they need, the right medical care—and things are progressing well. Having connected with thousands of parents (through my practice, speaking at live events, and through my websites), it's all too common for parents to feel that they're not getting the support they need. In this case they need to *advocate* for their child—to get the support that's necessary.

And every time a parent stands up for his or her child's needs, and advocates effectively, it's helping their own child, and it is actually paving the way for other individuals to benefit as well in the future.

It's not always easy to be the "trail blazer," but this is what often happens when parents need to stand up for their child's needs.

As I mentioned, some parents are reluctant about following the "ADD Parent's Journey," of going from student to expert to advocate.

The "job" of being the parent to an ADD child or teen can have its very challenging times. It can be tiring and thankless. And it can seem that one has to advocate and educate everywhere—even with "well meaning" family members. As a result, some parents feel too tired or burned out to want to be an expert or advocate.

In my experience, most parents are on the ADD Parent's Journey already—even if they are burned out and not wanting to be on it. If you're a parent of a child or teen with ADD, I encourage you to embrace this journey. Give yourself credit for the knowledge that you have (or are getting), the expertise you have and your ability to advocate.

Most of the time it's a path you're going to follow anyway… Why not choose to do it enthusiastically? (And give yourself credit for doing it well!).

CHAPTER 3

Step 1: Education about ADD

now we'll begin to cover the 7 Steps in the Attention Difference Disorder System. This is my approach to ensure that you cover all of the areas to help ADD and achieve a great outcome.

Step 1 is all about becoming educated about ADD.

Some people wonder why I put education as Step 1 before even covering the diagnosis of ADD.

The reason is simple. Before a child or teen gets a diagnosis of ADD— someone has to be concerned—aware—that ADD may be present. There has to be an "Index of Suspicion." People learn to suspect ADD in different ways.

The most common way that parents consider it in their child is because a teacher suggests that ADD may be present and asks them to see their doctor for assessment. Sometimes parents suspect it themselves, or they read an article or news story about it. And there are other possible routes, as well.

But even before getting a diagnosis, people need to learn about the condition and begin to understand what ADD is all about.

If you're reading this book *after* a diagnosis is made, then this chapter will share with you the facts you need to know, and the next chapter will help you to determine if a proper assessment was done, as well as help you to feel confident about the diagnosis itself.

If you don't have a diagnosis for your child or teen yet, and you just suspect ADD, then this chapter will give you facts that you need, and the next chapter will help you to ensure that you get a thorough assessment for ADD.

Why Education about ADD Is Critically Important

ADD is a condition which is generally present for years, not days, weeks or months. This means that when a child has it at six years of age, they almost certainly will still have it at 10 years of age, and 16 years of age. This means that kids and teens go through different developmental stages with their ADD. The issues which are a concern to the parent of a six year old will be different than the issues of that same parent when their child is 10 or 16 years old.

This is why it's very important to keep learning about ADD. Because once you feel that you've mastered it, your child will grow up, hit new developmental challenges and issues, and what was working before isn't working now. New problems arise, and new strategies are needed.

Additionally, the research on ADD continues. There are always new medication trials, new therapy trials, and new basic research which help us to deepen our understanding of the very nature of the condition.

How should you keep up to date with ADD?

I encourage you to start with the foundation in the subject that you'll receive in this book.

It's also important to rely on your healthcare professionals—i.e. the medical specialists who assess and monitor your child. Additionally, you should continue to rely on the other professionals involved: psychologists, teachers or special education support teachers, social workers, occupational therapists, etc. Each professional can contribute his or her area of expertise to your understanding of this condition.

I strongly encourage you to take part in parent support groups—especially if there is one that is local. When you're starting out, the other ADD parents are an outstanding resource for you. They often know of professionals in your community who can help you to get the resources you need, and they can share strategies which have worked for them. As you progress, you then become the expert helping the other parents.

You can also sign up for email updates from me at:

www.AttentionDifferenceDisorder.com/Bonus

Fact 1: ADD isn't New

Many people criticize this diagnosis, saying that it is just a creation of our modern society. People often believe that it is really an issue of the past two decades, where our society has become very "electronic" and fast paced. The reality is that there has been better recognition and understanding of ADD in our more recent times, and this has led to the appearance of an increase in diagnosis. Many people believe that the rates of ADD are spiralling out of control, when in fact good research shows that even at the current rates of diagnosis, there are many people with this condition who are not receiving a diagnosis and the treatment which could help them.

Dr. Russell Barkley, a leading researcher and author on ADHD, published in his ADHD Report in February 2009, that he had found an early medical document from a Scottish physician, dating back to 1798, describing the clinical presentation which today would be diagnosed as ADD. This shows there is at least over 200 years of history to the symptom pattern that we now call ADD.

In 1854, Dr. Heinrich Hoffman published the poem "Fidgety Phil" in which he clearly describes the hyperactivity which boys with ADD often display. He writes:

Let me see if Philip can

Be a little gentleman;

Let me see if he is able

To sit still for once at table:

Thus Papa bade Phil behave;

And Mamma looked very grave.

But fidgety Phil,

He won't sit still;

—*Dr. Heinrich Hoffman, The Story of Fidgety Phil*

In 1901, Dr. Still described in detail the clinical syndrome which we now call ADD. And, in 1937, Dr. Bradley was the first doctor who found that stimulant medication helped to treat ADD children.

As you can see, there is a long history of the medical profession being aware of the symptoms and condition we now call ADD, and a medication treatment for ADD discovered as well, long ago.

Fact 2: ADD is Real

Many wonder if ADD is real. It is said that it is just a collection of symptoms, and not a true medical condition. To address this question, we have to see if the diagnosis helps us in the way that we need it to. Does it help us to understand more about the challenges that the person with ADD will deal with, and help us to predict treatment responses and risks of not receiving treatment?

The answers are clearly "yes." With ADD, there is a clearly described set of symptoms, which have been well researched. We know that when individuals meet the criteria for diagnosis:

- They respond reasonably reliably to the researched treatments available for the condition;

- They are at higher risk of long term consequences if they don't receive treatment; and
- It often runs in their families – i.e. it is genetic;
- Recent brain research shows differences in brain function in particular regions in the case of those individuals who have ADD;
- And genetic research is finding "candidate genes" in those individuals, which are believed to be related to the underlying cause.

In short, ADD is real.

Fact 3: Social Issues Do Not Cause ADD

It's very common for people to read an article in a magazine or newspaper which says that ADD is caused by some kind of social issue.

People often say that ADD is caused by:

- violent video games;
- teachers who don't care enough about the students;
- parents who work too much and don't invest enough time with their kids;
- a loss of "family values" in our society;
- or a whole range of other "social issues."

The reality is that ADD is a real medical condition based on biology and neurobiology as well as genetics. There is no reliable scientific evidence that ADD has any social cause. There is, however, a significant body of research showing that the cause of ADD has a medical basis.

This issue gets tricky when social issues make ADD seem worse—which they can. Consider the example of a child with ADHD who has a single parent family where the parent works long hours to support the family. If the child attends a school where there are insufficient resources to support their particular needs, this can lead to a seemingly worse presentation, and it may seem that it is the cause of the ADD.

These factors in and of themselves, however, do not cause ADD. They may worsen it, but they don't cause it. And we know that there are many individuals who live in such circumstances, who do not meet the diagnostic criteria for ADD.

In summary, *social issues do not cause ADD*. They may worsen the presentation if an individual has ADD, but they don't cause it.

This is important for you to remember. The next time you read an article or have a "well-wishing" individual tell you that ADD is caused by violent movies (or some other social cause), you can inform them that in fact, ADD is a true medical condition. You can explain that while it may not be good for young kids to see violent movies, the violent movies do not cause ADD.

Fact 4: ADD is a Brain Based Disorder

It's fair to say that Psychiatry is a medical specialty which has been "behind the times" compared to other medical specialties. This is because it's been much easier to research other areas of the body for decades or even centuries. For example, in ancient Greece, if someone died clutching their chest, they could do an autopsy, and find the damage caused by a heart attack.

However, in psychiatry, the situation is different. If someone lived in ancient Greece, and they were forgetful, impulsive and got themselves into trouble (i.e. exhibited ADD symptoms) and they passed away—if an autopsy of their brain was done—they would see no difference from that of an individual, deceased, who had not exhibited that behavior. It has only been in the past couple of decades that the technology exists allowing us to truly begin to see what is going on in the brain *as it's functioning*. There are now "functional imaging" strategies that allow researchers to see which areas of the brain are used for different thinking functions. In recent years, we've been able to look at the differences in individuals with ADHD—how their brains work differently.

There is growing evidence that there are differences in the brains of individuals with ADD. The current medical literature shows that there are differences; it becomes apparent when a large group of individuals with ADD are compared to a group of (non-ADD) normal "controls." The science, however, is not yet at the stage where any one individual can have a brain scan to confirm or deny the existence of ADD.

The brain imaging research documents several areas of interest in the brain. These include areas such as the prefrontal cortex, the cerebellum, as well as several other brain regions. In the very recent past, there have been studies showing that *differences in brain functioning with ADD individuals are corrected with the use of ADD medications*!

This new research is very promising—promising to help show that ADD is real, a true medical condition, and that treatments can improve brain functioning. Images from brain-based research also help families to explain that ADD is a true medical condition—and that it is not just caused by social issues.

Does this mean that in fact individuals with ADHD have "brain damage" because their brains don't work properly?

Absolutely not! My interpretation is that the new brain research shows that there are *differences* in ADD individuals. While there have only been one or two studies which show that medications can balance these differences, it's my hope that in the future, studies will show that any kind of effective treatment actually helps the individual to rebalance their brain functioning. It is also my hope that we will get longer term studies about how treatments impact on these brain differences, because the current studies are only about short term treatment.

Fact 5: ADD Has Been Found At Similar Rates Across The World

Many people believe that ADD is a North American phenomenon. They suggest that it is the demands of our fast-paced Western society that lead to the high rates of diagnosis of ADD. Or even worse—they suggest that the well developed system of pharmaceutical company marketing has led to the false over-recognition of ADD in North America.

There have been many epidemiological studies done all over the world. Epidemiological studies are community-based studies looking at the rate of the diagnosis in a particular community. There have been studies done on multiple continents, with different cultures, in different languages. The general summary is that ADD occurs approximately five to seven percent of the time in school-age children. This is a consistent finding across different cultures and different parts of the world.

In other words, ADD is not a North American phenomenon. It has been found around the world at similar rates, despite very different regions and very different cultures.

Fact 6: ADD Runs in Families

ADD has been shown to be a genetic disorder. Twin studies document that ADD is approximately 80 to 85 percent heritable. This means that the majority of the reasons for an individual developing ADD relates specifically to genetics.

In my experience, it's been very common for a parent to start reading about ADD when the child has been diagnosed, and realize that they themselves, or their spouse, either has the condition or has significant ADD traits. It is also common for a cousin, sibling or other family member to also have ADD when a child is diagnosed.

When I'm assessing a child for ADD, I'll admit that I always wonder if one or the other parent may have ADD traits or the full disorder. Some parents are open to this kind of discussion and others are not. When a family is not particularly open to the idea of considering the possibility that one of the parents may have ADD, I take a gentler approach. I generally ask which parent the child's personality is most like. This can often be an opening to the discussion of whether a parent may have ADD traits.

It's quite important to consider whether a parent may have ADD or ADD traits. This becomes increasingly important when treatment recommendations are made to help the child with ADD. Treatment for ADD often involves parents establishing structure and support for their child. Certain things need to be done routinely, i.e. coordinate with the school, set up homework routines, take medication at a certain time, etc.

If a parent is struggling with ADD himself, it can often be hard for him to maintain the structure that he needs to help his child, and to implement the recommendations as needed. Thus, it is quite important to review whether in fact mom or dad have ADD or ADD traits. And if they do, it is important for them to seek help both for themselves and for their family members who depend on them.

Fact 7: Not All ADD Is Genetic

We've covered the fact that ADD is approximately 80 percent heritable. What about the other 20 percent? What causes that?

As a group, these are called the "acquired" cases of ADD. In other words, they appear because of something that happened, rather than from genetics. We can split the acquired causes into two groups: prenatal (i.e. before birth) and postnatal (i.e. after birth).

The prenatal causes of ADD include:

- Maternal smoking during pregnancy;
- Maternal drinking alcohol during pregnancy;
- Prematurity of birth.

Each of these causes increases the risks of developing ADD, but it is not certain that if a mother smokes during pregnancy that the child will have ADD.

The postnatal causes of ADD include:

- Head injuries;
- Lead poisoning when young (i.e. 0 to 3 years old);

- Survival from acute lymphoblastic leukemia (ALL) —the chemotherapy often induces ADD.

If your child has had one of these risk factors, then it is worth discussing with your doctor. Sometimes, the acquired cases of ADD don't respond as well to treatment—including medication.

Fact 8: Do More Boys Have ADD Than Girls?

If you ask people about what they picture in their minds when they hear "ADD," most people envision a young boy who runs around too much and is too hyperactive. And this "stereotype" goes far beyond people's general perception. At this time, the medical profession generally diagnoses three or four times as many boys with ADD as we do for every girl with ADD.

If we look at the gender difference in adult ADD, what new research is showing is that the male to female ratio is equal. This means that there is one male to one female in adult ADD.

Since we know that ADD is a developmental disorder— i.e. it starts in childhood—this means that these women with ADD aren't just starting to develop ADD later in life ... they are in fact just not diagnosed or "picked up" when they are kids.

Why is there such a discrepancy between boys and girls in childhood?

The rate of diagnosis of ADD and boys is much higher for several reasons. Firstly, boys tend to have much more hyperactivity with their ADD whereas girls tend to have much more inattention. This means that boys are noticed quite readily by parents and teachers as needing help. And girls with inattention who day dream too much, don't often get the attention of the adults in their lives.

Additionally, it's very common for boys to have behavioral problems with their ADD such as oppositional defiant disorder or conduct disorder, whereas girls tend to have more emotional issues. These behavioral issues lead to boys being recognized more often than girls because they cause much more disruption.

While it's very important we identify and support the boys, it's even more critically important that we find the girls who have difficulties with ADD. It is important that we identify them early, so they can get the support they need, and allow them to progress forward and achieve the potential that they are able to achieve.

The issues described above can be described in this way—there is a referral bias. In other words, several factors increase the likelihood that boys will be referred for assessment by a mental health or medical professional, whereas several factors decrease the likelihood that girls will be referred for assessment. Thus, there is a referral bias.

In summary, boys and girls likely have ADD at the same rate, however we need to do a better job of identifying that the girls have ADD and getting them help earlier.

Fact 9: ADD Can Last Past the Teenage Years

ADD has been thought to be a childhood disorder for years. It was routine medical practice to say that ADD ended at 18 years old—that is until approximately the mid-1990s. There were some pioneering researchers who followed groups of kids and teens with ADD into their adult life, and they were able to establish that many people still have ADD when they're adults.

Current research suggests that approximately 60 to 70 percent of kids or teens with ADD will still have it as adults.

This is one of the reasons that it's critically important to get a full, comprehensive approach put in place to help support kids and teens with ADD. If we can help them to turn their deficits into differences and their differences into strengths, we can actually help to prepare young people with ADD for a productive adult life—whether they still have the disorder are not.

Fact 10: ADD Can Impact a Lot More Than School

It used to be a standard recommendation that ADD medication be given just for school days. The stimulant medicines are unique in that they can be taken just for the days they are needed. Hence, people would not take medication on weekends, nor would they take medication on school holidays or summer breaks.

The basic assumption was that the medication was aiding academics and that's all it was needed for.

For the fast past 15 years or so, researchers in ADD have established that ADD has a much broader impact than just academics. In fact, ADD impacts many areas of an individual's life. The areas impacted include: social relationships, emotional functioning, psychological growth and development, self-esteem, and much more.

In other words, when an individual's ADD medication was stopped for weekends and holidays, he or she was not getting the benefit of being able to function well while interacting in the numerous non-academic areas that they were functioning in. This was ultimately a disservice to patients with ADD.

Current recommendations are to take medication seven days per week throughout the year. Certainly there are some circumstances where you and your doctor may make a decision otherwise, however the general recommendation at this time is to treat ADD without interruption.

There is new research being done on quality of life and ADD, documenting the belief that, when ADD is well treated, it does improve functioning in social, emotional and psychological areas as well as academic or occupational areas.

Fact 11: There are Significant Risks to Untreated ADD

As we will cover in Step 2, one of the critical parts of the diagnosis is the fact that there is impairment from the ADD symptoms. Impairment refers to negative consequences in your child or teen's life because of the ADD symptoms. Long term research has shown that untreated ADD can lead to a variety of different consequences, many of which can be quite severe.

With untreated ADD, there are risks for problems like:

- **Academic underachievement:** Kids and teens with ADD often do worse than they are capable of doing in school. Over many years, this can lead to lower grades, and ultimately not going as far in school as a student is capable of going. This leads to a lower level of employment than might have been possible otherwise.

- **Occupational functioning:** Teens (and adults) with ADD often are underemployed—i.e. not working up to their potential. They often earn less than they could be for their position.

- **Accidents and injuries:** ADD kids and teens are at higher risks of accidents and injuries. Many studies have shown that there are increase healthcare costs in untreated ADD kids/teens.

- **Substance abuse:** Kids and teens with untreated ADD are at higher risk of drug and alcohol problems. This is covered in more detail in Step 7: Treatment Integration.

- **Sexual behavior:** There are higher risks of teenage pregnancy, as well as sexually transmitted infections (just think—ADD impulsivity, and then add in teenage hormones...).

- **Criminality:** Kids and teens with untreated ADD are much more likely to get arrested at least once. If you take all teens who get arrested once, the ADD teens are much more likely to get arrested a second time.

- **Social functioning:** Kids and teens with untreated ADD often struggle socially. They may not perceive well enough what is going on with their friends, and then they can become isolated. Unfortunately, the gap grows over the years—i.e. as social interactions become more complicated with age (i.e. life is a lot more complicated for 16 year olds than it is for six year olds), ADD kids can have an even greater struggle.

- **Driving:** Teens with ADD who drive are at higher risk of motor vehicle accidents and traffic citations. This is an area of ADD which is a significant public health issue and can actually be lethal—knowing that motor vehicle accidents is one of the top killers of teenagers, and knowing that ADD teens can be inattentive behind the wheel—this is a very important issue for safety. (I strongly encourage parents to set very strict guidelines around driving with ADD teens—maybe even requiring medication to allow the teen to get the keys.)

The bottom line: Without good treatment, kids and teens with ADD are at risk for many different problems. Although only driving can be lethal, the cumulative effect of all of the possible different problems can have a big impact on your child's long-term prospects. Often times, each challenge can build onto another, and there can be a "downward negative spiral." While strategies can help you get out of a downward spiral, it is far better to avoid it entirely by intervening early.

Fact 12: The Diagnosis of ADD Can Be Missed For Years

ADD is a developmental disorder. This means that it's in the brain and it starts being an issue in childhood, whether it is diagnosed in childhood or not.

Therefore, some may wonder: "Why is ADD often diagnosed in adolescence (or even in adulthood), if it starts in childhood?"

There are many factors which can interfere with an individual getting the diagnosis of ADD early in life.

The first factor to consider: some people may not even consider the possibility. If the doctor, teachers, parents or any other individuals involved in the child's life don't consider that ADD is a possibility, then it certainly will not be diagnosed. With increased awareness of this condition, hopefully this will become less of an issue with time.

Another factor to consider is the fact that the severity of the ADD symptoms has an impact on whether ADD is diagnosed. In other words, if an individual has very severe symptoms, it's much more likely that they'll be recognized earlier in life. If they have very mild symptoms, it's much more likely they will go many years before anyone picks up on it.

The amount of support available can impact the rate of diagnosis as well. Some kids go to a small school, where there are a lot of supports and structure around the children. When this happens, the ADD symptoms may not be as apparent. This could also delay the recognition of the condition.

Intellect can play a big factor as well. In other words, if the child is quite bright, with a high IQ, parents and teachers may not pick up on the fact that they have ADD. They're still getting B's and C's—though parents and teachers know they could do much better if they only "apply themselves." Then the discussion of "willpower" and the need to "apply oneself" becomes the discussion rather than looking for ADD as the possible cause.

As a professional clinician, working in my office, I often look for the "transitional years" in school to find the symptoms coming out and becoming more of a concern. By this I mean there are significant changes in expectations when a child goes from elementary school to middle school, and from middle school to high school. For example, in high school, a child needs to keep much more organized, stay on top of things, and deal with multiple demands in a way that wasn't necessary in the earlier school years. If the child was doing well in his or her early years of school and starts to do poorly in 9th grade, I certainly consider ADD as a possibility, and look for aspects of ADD which were present but unrecognized earlier on.

If symptoms are just showing up in 9th grade, this may be an indication that the individual's coping strategies, intellect and other factors can no longer compensate for their symptoms of ADD.

Other transitional times to look for include transition to college or university, or entering the workforce. If ADD symptoms become apparent at that stage of life, the clinician needs to consider the possibility that there have been ADD symptoms all along, which were compensated for and thus the ADD wasn't recognized.

Watch for certain "key words." When I'm seeing a teen or young adult, and the parent keeps saying certain words, it makes me consider the possibility of ADD. These words are said extremely commonly when ADD is there and it hasn't been recognized. These words include:

- **Lazy:** "He's just lazy."
- **Unmotivated:** "He just can't get motivated to do well."
- **Moments of brilliance:** "When he is "on" he can do brilliant work—it just happens infrequently."
- **Apply himself:** If he would just "apply himself"; "He can do great work when he tries."
- **Potential:** "He could do such great things if he just lived up to his potential."

These "key words" do not diagnose ADD on their own. When I hear them, I just consider them small "red flags" that make my ears prick up and consider ADD as a possibility. Remember—to diagnose ADD at all, one has to consider it as a possibility. The medical term for this is having an "Index of

Suspicion." When a teen comes to see me with a complaint around depression or anxiety, and there are issues around school (which there often are when there's depression or anxiety), and I hear one of these keywords—I strongly consider ADD as a possibility. In the example of a depressed or anxious teen, I would stabilize and treat the depression and anxiety first and then spend time assessing for ADD.

In my experience, the word "potential" is often used so much, that teens with undiagnosed ADD have a strong, negative association with it. If I even say the word it gets them to roll their eyes and have an emotional reaction to it. Recently a teen in my office said (while rolling his eyes), "If I had a dime for every time I've heard that…" Although many parents of teens may talk about their teens not achieving their potential, when a teen has undiagnosed ADD it is far more prevalent and pervasive an issue.

Fact 13: ADD Rarely Comes Alone

It is very common for kids and teens with ADD to have at least one other psychiatric disorder diagnosed as well. The medical term for this is *co-morbidity*. This refers to the fact that the additional diagnosis (or diagnoses) increase the "morbidity," or suffering that the individual experiences. As a doctor who works with a lot of kids and teens with ADD, I prefer to call these "co-existing" conditions—because families have to deal with enough negativity to begin with.

While co-existing conditions will be discussed in great depth in Step 7 of the "Attention Difference Disorder System: Treatment Integration," I'll give a brief introduction here.

The frequency of co-existing conditions is 75 percent in kids and teens with ADD. That means that only 25 percent of kids and teens with ADD have "simple ADD." The rest have ADD which is complicated by one or more disorders.

Table 1 provides an overview of the common co-existing conditions with ADD in kids and teens:

Coexisting Condition:	Approximate Rate:
Oppositional Defiant Disorder	Up to 60 percent
Learning Disabilities	Up to 40 percent
Depression	Up to 35 percent
Anxiety Disorders	Up to 45 percent
Conduct Disorder	Up to 25 percent
Substance Abuse/dependence	Up to 30 percent

Table 2: ADD and the rates of co-existing conditions in kids and teens

Please note that this doesn't add up to 100 percent because some kids may have two or three co-existing disorders.

The main takeaway about co-existing conditions is this: Often times the co-existing condition has a big impact on the treatment and outcome for the child with ADD. In other words, a child with ADD plus Anxiety often has different challenges and treatment needs than a child with ADD and a behavior disorder. The specifics about this topic will be covered in more depth when we get to Step 7: Treatment Integration. We need to build the foundation for ADD treatment before we get into the adjustments needed for co-existing conditions.

Fact 14: ADD is Thought to be a Disorder of Executive Functioning

When we diagnose ADD, we use the diagnostic criteria of the American Psychiatric Association's Diagnostic and Statistical Manual (known as the DSM-IV-TR). These criteria list the symptoms of ADD (officially called AD/HD) which a clinician can use to diagnose the condition. The DSM is a manual which describes symptoms and the researched diagnostic criteria—but doesn't discuss what actually causes the condition.

Newer research in the field of ADD point to ADD being caused by a disorder in *executive functions.*

Executive functions refer to the cognitive (thinking) processes that allow us to plan, prioritize and organize. They are the highest level of thinking.

When thinking about the executive functions, I often think about the movie *Air Force One.* In this film, Harrison Ford plays the US President, and his airplane (Air Force One) is hijacked by terrorists. Glenn Close plays the Vice-President, and she is sitting at a board room table with all of her military advisors and experts as they plan out what they can do to help the president. This "board room" has experts from many areas, each being skilled at his/her area. For example, the director of the Air Force has resources at his disposal, and the director of the Navy has resources at his disposal, etc. In this albeit fictional example, the ability for this "team" to achieve its goal involves the absolute necessity for the team to work together and coordinate well. It doesn't matter how expert the air force is—if they work out of coordination with the rest of the team, then their efforts will work against the overall achievement of the goal.

The executive functions of the brain are analogous to the board room table or "team" in the example described above. It is the brain's planning center. Even if the brain is good at certain functions, if they are done out of order, or without coordination, then they are considered ineffective. One could argue that Harrison Ford would not have been saved if the "board room table team" didn't work together to ensure its success. If everyone did what they thought was best on their own, there wouldn't be a good team, and the outcome could have been mayhem.

Executive functions are described and defined differently in many texts. That said, most researchers and doctors agree on the basic executive functions. There are different scales and tools used to measure executive functions. One such tool is the BRIEF®—the Behavior Rating Inventory of Executive Functioning. It is used in ADHD research studies to look at the executive functioning of the participants. I consider it a big advancement in the field of ADHD that executive functions are starting to be measured in regular research trials.

Although there are many different definitions and classifications of executive functioning, the BRIEF® questionnaire can be used to look at the areas of executive functioning. The BRIEF® breaks executive functions into the following scales (and a brief description follows each concept):

- **Inhibit:** This refers to the ability to control impulses; stop behavior.
- **Shift:** The ability to move freely from one activity/situation to another; transition; problem-solve flexibly.
- **Emotional Control:** The ability to modulate emotional responses appropriately.
- **Initiate:** The ability to begin activity; generate ideas.
- **Working Memory:** The ability to hold information in mind for purpose of completing a task.
- **Plan/Organize:** The ability to anticipate future events; set goals; develop steps; grasp main ideas.
- **Monitor:** The ability to check work; assess one's own performance.

It's important for you to understand what executive functioning is, and to begin to understand the impact that executive functions have on functioning in ADD. In other words, if someone has "improved" (or "high functioning") executive functions, then they generally have a better outcome than if they are "poor functioning" with their executive functions. The tricky thing is that even with improved core symptoms of ADD, there can still be deficits in executive functioning that can be a real issue for people, and cause ongoing impairment.

Talk to an expert in ADD about your child or teen's executive functions. Most child psychiatrists and paediatricians who are experts in ADD can have a good discussion with you about executive functioning. Psychologists are likely the best experts to discuss executive functioning with you—especially to discuss your child's specific strengths and weaknesses and strategies which may help you to improve executive functioning in your child.

Other resources to consider include these two books: *Smart but Scattered* by Dawson and Guare, and *Late, Lazy and Unprepared* by Cooper-Kahn and Dietzel.

Fact 15: Use ADD as an Explanation, not an Excuse

There are many people who become concerned about how the medical profession is diagnosing conditions in a way which seem to absolve people of their responsibility for their actions. With ADD, the concern is that kids or teens will be considered to have too much impulsivity or inattention—so how can we expect them to control their behavior?

In my clinical practice, I have seen kids and teens that have become "wise" to this. After their parent educates others about the fact that they have ADD, the child tries to make sure that others lower their expectations of him, in order that that his ADD becomes the excuse for why people shouldn't expect much from him.

In my experience and opinion, this is actually very harmful for the individual with ADD.

Having ADD can allow you to understand what may be contributing to a specific challenge. It helps to provide an explanation. And as you review the possible explanation(s) for the challenge, you can find solutions for each of those issues. Whereas if one uses ADD as an excuse—there is no practical solution developed, based on the fact that it is considered to be just the ADD.

For example, if a boy with ADD struggles in his after-school program with fighting for toys with another child—if we use ADD as an excuse, the only remedy we have is to say, "Oh well, this is going to happen, because he has ADD."

If we use ADD as an explanation, then we look at the specific challenges going on, and see if we can then find remedies. For example, perhaps that is a time that the medication is wearing off. Or maybe he hasn't had a chance to get some physical exercise for hours. As we look at how the ADD can impact his functioning, and contribute to the challenge (i.e. we use ADD as an explanation), then we can actually begin to find solutions for the problems.

Now that you know some of the fundamental facts about ADD, let's move on to Step 2—ensuring that you have a proper assessment for ADD.

CHAPTER 4

Step 2: Ensuring a Proper Assessment and Diagnosis of ADD

O ne of the biggest challenges that people have when they're getting started with ADD is being certain about the diagnosis itself. Parents often wonder if their child was diagnosed properly, and if the "proper testing" was done. Well-meaning friends and family can erode a parent's confidence in the diagnosis when they suggest that all kids have some degree of inattention, or hyperactivity. When it comes to considering treatments like medication, it is very important to be sure about the diagnosis.

ADD is diagnosed using criteria which are published by the American Psychiatric Association in the *Diagnostic and Statistical Manual, 4th Edition*, Text Revision (DSM-IV-TR). There are other diagnostic systems—including the International Classification of Diseases and Related Health Problems—10th Revision (ICD-10)[1]. In North America, and many other areas, the DSM is used as the standard and will be discussed in this text.

---

1   In the ICD-10, ADHD has a different name; it is called: Hyperkinetic Disorder.

The DSM-IV-TR criteria for ADHD are reproduced below.

Attention-Deficit/Hyperactivity Disorder Criterion

A. Either **(1)** or **(2)**:

(1) Six (or more) of the following symptoms of **inattention** have persisted for at least six months to a degree that is maladaptive and inconsistent with developmental level:

Inattention:

(a) Often fails to give close attention to details or makes careless mistakes in schoolwork, work or other activities.

(b) Often has difficulty sustaining attention in tasks or play activities.

(c) Often does not seem to listen when spoken to directly.

(d) Often does not follow through on instructions and fails to finish schoolwork, chores, or duties in the workplace (not due to oppositional behavior or failure to understand instructions).

(e) Often has difficulty organizing tasks and activities.

(f) Often avoids, dislikes, or is reluctant to engage in tasks that require sustained mental effort (such as school work or home work).

(g) Often loses things necessary for tasks and activities (e.g. toys, school assignments, pencils, books or tools).

(h) Is often easily distracted by extraneous stimuli.

(i) Is often forgetful in daily activities.

(2) Six (or more) of the following symptoms of **hyperactivity-impulsivity** have persisted for at least six months to a degree that is maladaptive and inconsistent with developmental level:

Hyperactivity:

    (a) Often fidgets with hands or feet or squirms in seat.

    (b) Often leaves seat in classroom or in other situations in which remaining seated is expected.

    (c) Often runs about or climbs excessively in situations in which it is inappropriate (in adolescents or adults, may be limited to subjective feelings of restlessness).

    (d) Often has difficulty playing or engaging in leisure activities quietly.

    (e) Is often "on the go" or often acts as if "driven by a motor."

    (f) Often talks excessively.

Impulsivity:

    (g) Often blurts out answers before questions have been completed.

    (h) Often has difficulty awaiting turn.

    (i) Often interrupts or intrudes on others (e.g. butts into conversations or games).

B. Some hyperactive-impulsive or inattentive symptoms that caused impairment were present before age seven years.

C. Some impairment from the symptoms is present in two or more settings (e.g., at school [or work] and at home).

D. There must be clear evidence of clinically significant impairment in social, academic, or occupational functioning.

E. The symptoms do not occur exclusively during the course of a Pervasive Developmental Disorder, Schizophrenia, or other Psychotic Disorder and are not better accounted for by another mental disorder (e.g. Mood Disorder, Anxiety Disorder, Dissociative Disorder, or a Personality Disorder).

Code Based on Type:

314.01 Attention-Deficit/Hyperactivity Disorder, Combined Type: if both criteria A1 and A2 are met for the past six months

314.00 Attention-Deficit/Hyperactivity Disorder, Predominantly Inattentive Type: if Criterion A1 is met but Criterion A2 is not met for the past six months

314.01 Attention-Deficit/Hyperactivity Disorder, Predominantly Hyperactive-Impulsive Type: if Criterion A2 is met but Criterion A1 is not met for the past six months

Coding Note: For individuals (especially adolescents and adults) who currently have symptoms that no longer meet full criteria, "In Partial Remission" should be specified.

Reprinted with permission from the Diagnostic and Statistical Manual of Mental Disorders, Fourth Edition, Text Revision, (Copyright 2000). American Psychiatric Association.

When looking at the DSM criteria, you'll notice several important factors which are important in the diagnosis of ADD. These are described and elaborated on below:

1) There are nine symptoms of inattention, and to meet the diagnosis, one has to have six out of nine symptoms (or more).

2) There are nine symptoms of hyperactivity/impulsivity, and to meet the diagnosis, one has to have six out of nine symptoms (or more).

3) The symptoms have to be present for more than six months. Generally speaking, unless a child is quite young, there is a history of these symptoms for years or months, rather than weeks.

4) The symptoms have to be at a level which is more than expected for their developmental level. In other words, we don't expect a six year old to

concentrate as well as a 10 year old. The expert assessing for ADD will have a sense of what is expected for your child's developmental level. Many parents and teachers have a good sense of this as well.

5) The symptoms have to be present in two or more settings. This is important to ensure that the symptoms are in the individual, and not just due to one setting. In other words, if the symptoms are present only at school, but never at home, never at soccer games, never at an after school program—then it suggests that there is a problem at school, not a problem with the individual. When we can establish that the symptoms are present in two or more settings, this suggests that it is truly the individual, not just the particular setting.

6) The symptoms must cause impairment. The impairment can be in the realms of: social, emotional, psychological, academic or occupational functioning. In other words, the child or teen is not functioning up to the level that they are able to, because the ADD symptoms are interfering. Impairment is a critical factor to the diagnosis of ADD. ***Without impairment, there isn't a diagnosis.*** Impairment is why the symptoms are a concern, and why treatment needs to be considered. In my office, if medication is considered for ADD and parents are concerned about making the decision—the main point to review in making the decision is the extent of the impairment in their child. When there is significant impairment, it is worth considering medication and all treatment options available.

7) There are symptoms present before the age of seven years. This is important particularly for older teens or adults who are being assessed for ADD. This criterion is present to ensure that there are symptoms present for a long time. Since ADD is a developmental disorder—meaning that it starts in childhood—there have to be symptoms present early on to

ensure that it is truly ADD. If the ADD symptoms start later in life, then it is not truly ADD. The doctor would need to look for other possible explanations, like Depression, Anxiety, PTSD, substance abuse, etc.

8) The ADD symptoms are not caused by another disorder. This final criterion is present to help ensure that the inattention and hyperactivity/impulsivity are actually due to the ADD and not something else. If, for example, the inattention has only occurred during the course of a depression, then it would not be ADD. If, however, the ADD symptoms pre-date the depression, then an individual could have both ADD and depression. We will spend more time on co-existing conditions in Step 7: Treatment Integration.

9) The DSM-IV-TR documents three official diagnoses:
    1) **AD/HD predominantly Inattentive Type**: This is the diagnosis when six out of nine symptoms (or more) of inattention are present, but the hyperactive-impulsive symptoms are not at that level.
    2) **AD/HD predominantly Hyperactive Impulsive Type:** This is the diagnosis when six out of nine symptoms (or more) of the hyperactivity impulsivity criteria are met, but the inattentive symptoms are not at that level.
    3) **AD/HD Combined Type**: This is the diagnosis when the criteria for both inattentive and hyperactive/impulsive criteria are met.

As we've discussed previously, for the purposes of this book, we will use the name: ADD—referring to the differences in AD/HD, rather than the deficits.

How to Get Assessed for ADD

To get assessed for ADD, most people start with their Family Doctor or Primary Care Physician. Even if this doctor is not an expert in ADD, he or she generally knows who in your community has that expertise and who can help you out. Generally, this is an easy first step. You book an appointment, go see the doctor and explain that you are concerned about the possibility of ADD (or you discuss the concerns that the school shared, etc.). The doctor, most of the time, points you in the right direction, and you are on your way to getting an expert assessment for the diagnosis of ADD.

Sometimes, the first step doesn't work so easily. There are some Primary Care doctors who don't know enough about ADD, and they may say something like: "Oh, your daughter is fine. Just tell her to try harder, and everything will be OK." This is where it can be frustrating for parents—because it is hard enough to have to fight the stigma in society at large, and even harder when you have to fight the stigma that your own doctor has! If you end up in a situation like this, I strongly encourage you to find a local ADD parent support group. The parents you meet there can let you know which doctors in your community can help, and give you some advice on how to get support and resources in your community. If you can't access a parent support group, see if the helpful staff at your child's school may know of a doctor who has helped other students with ADD, or an ADD assessment.

After starting with your Primary Care Doctor—where do you go next?

There are a small number of Primary Care Doctors who have expertise in ADD—in which case they would do the assessment themselves. There aren't that many, but it is possible. Otherwise, you will often be referred to a Pediatrician, Child and Adolescent Psychiatrist, Neurologist, or Psychologist. There may be other professionals in your state or community who are licensed to diagnose, though most people will see one of the professionals mentioned.

It's best if you can get someone with expertise in ADD. Remember, it is OK for you to ask your doctor who is the local ADD expert, and to request to see that doctor. It is also alright to contact the specialist's office (that you are referred to) and ask them if the doctor has expertise in ADD.

And then after being on a waiting list for some time, you get to go for your assessment.

What to Expect At the ADD Assessment

Many ADD experts will ask you to come to your appointment with some "homework" done first. By this I mean that you may be asked to get some symptom checklists completed, and you may be asked to bring in copies of old report cards (going back as far as you have them), and copies of any psychological or educational testing which has been done, and any other reports which have been written. If your doctor's office didn't ask for you to bring these, it's probably still a good idea to bring them, and then things may go more smoothly and quickly.

When you go for the assessment, you can expect that the doctor will talk with your child/teen as well as yourself. When assessing for ADD it's important to get information from multiple people—so the doctor may want to talk to the school or other care providers. At the minimum, the doctor will likely ask for ADD symptom checklists to be completed by the other adults who supervise or observe your child/teen regularly.

Many Child Psychiatrists will book one hour for the initial assessments, and then bring you back to discuss the symptoms, diagnosis and treatment options at another appointment. Many Pediatricians book their offices differently, so they may have shorter appointments, and you may see them on more occasions to make the diagnosis and create the treatment plan. Psychologists often do more formal "testing" and they may have longer appointments. No matter how the appointments are booked, the assessment will have the same components.

At the core of it, ADD is a clinical diagnosis. That means it is diagnosed by clinicians, based on a clinical assessment (a clinician is the health professional that you see in the office, or "clinic"). The doctor will take a "history," meaning that he or she will listen to your concerns and issues, and then ask a whole range of clarifying questions. The doctor will ask questions about the core ADD symptoms, as well as about any other possible areas of concern—i.e. mood and anxiety symptoms, etc. The doctor will also inquire about how any symptoms discussed impact on your child or teen's functioning. The doctor will also review past medical history, past psychiatric history, family history of any psychiatric disorders, school history, as well as the current social circumstances for your family (i.e. parent's employment, living situations, any recent stressors in the family, etc.).

Even though many people would like to have a test for ADD, it's important for you to realize that there are no reliable tests to diagnose ADD. There is no blood test, no brain scan, or EEG machine which can reliably diagnose ADD. While there are many clinics where tests are marketed to diagnose ADD—there is little scientific research to back up the use of these tests. Often times, you are spending money on testing which will not really make much of a difference in your child's assessment or treatment. When looking at any test or treatment—you also need to look at the risks and benefits. When there is a brain scan involved, then your child is being exposed to radiation. When you consider the fact that there is no reliable science to back up the use of the test—the exposure to radiation is completely unnecessary, and the benefit from the test is not worth the risks of being exposed to radiation.

Remember—ADD is a clinical diagnosis, so it is diagnosed clinically—i.e. the old-fashioned way. That means we ask the questions, we go through the information, and we figure it out. And even though many people feel that this is a "lesser" approach than many other areas of medicine, when you look critically at diagnosis in medicine, even in the physical areas of medicine, it is generally accepted that 80 to 90 percent of any diagnosis is established based on the history taken, and the symptoms described. The physical exam and any tests ordered just help to confirm the doctor's impressions based on the history taken.

In ADD (and all psychiatric assessments), we do a "mental status examination," which includes observing the thought process, language, speech, movements, mood and affect, insight and judgment, etc. This is analogous to the physical exam in other areas of medicine and helps to establish the diagnosis as well. Although we don't order tests, we get collateral information (i.e. from other sources) and checklists completed to gather more complete information.

Is There Any Role for Physical Testing?

When assessing for ADD, it is important to ensure that certain physical issues aren't causing the ADD symptoms. For example, poor hearing or vision could lead to symptoms which appear to be inattention. It's fair to say that all kids going for an ADD assessment should get their hearing and vision checked. It would be awful to treat a child with ADD medication when they really need a hearing aid or eye-glasses.

When it comes to blood tests, sometimes they play an important role. Most of the scientific treatment guidelines do not recommend routine screening blood tests for kids and teens being assessed for ADD. What they do recommend is blood tests for any child or teen when there is a reason, based on the history or physical examination, to order blood tests. In other words, if the doctor is concerned about anemia, then ordering an iron/hemoglobin is reasonable; or if the doctor is concerned about thyroid functioning, then a test would be ordered to rule that out.

Some lab tests your doctor may consider:

- Hemoglobin to ensure there is no anemia.
- Thyroid Stimulating Hormone—to ensure that the thyroid isn't overactive (which can lead to increased energy, and agitation), or underactive (which can lead to decreased energy, less concentration and fatigue).
- Vitamin B12—if there is excessive fatigue.
- Liver and kidney functioning.
- Lead testing—if the child is in an environment with peeling lead paint.

Remember, ultimately your doctor will decide which blood tests can be helpful in your child's case. Talk to your doctor and ask questions to ensure that you understand your doctor's rationale for the testing (or lack thereof).

Another potentially helpful test is a sleep study. For a sleep study, the patient goes to a sleep lab and gets hooked up to the lab equipment and goes to bed. The lab monitors breathing and movements during sleep, as well as EEG monitoring to see that the brain is getting into the different stages of sleep in an appropriate way. One main concern in sleep is sleep apnea. This occurs when an individual snores excessively, and can actually have periods of stopping breathing during the night. Although the most common cause of this in older teens and adults is obesity—i.e. the thickened neck with weight can cause problems breathing in sleep—in younger kids, enlarged tonsils and adenoids can lead to sleep apnea as well. The sleep lab will also look for "restless leg syndrome."

One caution around sleep studies—some sleep labs have limited experience working with children and teens. Before going to a sleep lab (if you and your doctor decide that it is needed), call the lab and ask if they have experience with children and teens. If they don't, it is likely better to travel to a pediatric hospital or pediatric sleep lab to get a specialty assessment, even if it is a distance away. To be clear, sleep studies are NOT part of a routine ADD assessment, but may be added if your doctor is concerned about sleep issues.

A Special Note about EKG's

When we go into more depth about ADD medications in Step 5 of our system, you'll learn more about the cardiovascular side effects of the ADD medications. As a short summary—these medicines can increase heart rate and blood pressure a little bit. If there are no cardiac concerns (i.e. holes in the heart, or other such structural heart problems, or irregular heartbeats/arrhythmias), then the cardiovascular risks of ADD medications are very low.

There has been some scientific debate in the literature about whether an EKG is needed in everyone who takes an ADD medication. The American Cardiology Association came out with the directive that all children, teens and adults should have an EKG prior to using (and while using) ADD medications. However, after their papers on the subject appeared, the American Academy of Pediatrics came out saying that routine EKG's aren't needed.

Do I order EKG's for everyone? No, I don't. If there is any reason to do one, then I discuss it with the family and order one.

One advantage of EKG's is that they are non–invasive (i.e. the lab just puts sticky leads on the chest); they are quick and relatively inexpensive. But they aren't needed routinely.

Bringing the Diagnosis Together

After you and your doctor have gathered all of the information needed to complete the assessment, your doctor will take some time to explain the nature of the diagnosis, and his or her rationale for making the diagnosis. The doctor should tell you (or be able to tell, if you ask) which subtype of ADD your child has—i.e. inattentive only, hyperactive/impulsive only, or combined type.

It is also important for you to have a discussion with the doctor to understand the nature of the impairment that the doctor is concerned about. In other words, in the doctor's opinion, what are the areas of biggest impairment: school, family, social, psychological, etc.?

At the end of an assessment, doctors generally have a sense of the severity of the ADD in any particular patient. The severity of ADD (and most conditions) is generally considered either mild, moderate or severe. Ask your doctor which level your child's ADD is at. In my experience, if someone has a severe ADD, then my recommendations for treatment are different than if the ADD is mild. This refers to the fact that if the ADD is mild, then it is OK to take more time to decide on the treatments that are needed. However, if the ADD is severe, the consequences of the condition are significant and the impact is being experienced daily. It is better to make a quick decision about treatment and begin implementation as soon as possible.

The discussion with your doctor about the diagnosis of ADD should move quickly into a discussion about the treatment options for ADD.

Consider the components of the assessment of your child or teen. Did it have all of the components listed above? Are you content that he or she has been diagnosed thoroughly? If not, make a list of questions or issues that you'd like to ask your doctor about.

If your child has had all of the components necessary to make the diagnosis of ADD, then you need to accept that this is the diagnosis. Ask questions if you need to, and then begin to move toward treatment. And this takes us to the next step in the Attention Difference Disorder System, Step 3: Parenting Strategies for ADD.

CHAPTER 5

Step 3: Parenting Strategies for ADD

Parenting strategies for ADD are very important, and are really a cornerstone of the treatment of ADD in kids and teens. This is one of the most critical steps in the Attention Difference Disorder System for ADD—and this is why it comes right after the diagnosis.

Unfortunately, discussing parenting issues with parents of kids and teens with ADD can be a touchy issue as well. This relates to a long history of parent-blaming in the fields of mental health and psychiatry.

For decades (or longer), doctors trained in psychiatry and psychotherapy blamed parents for problems in their children. And, unfortunately, it was mostly the mothers. When anyone is thinking about psychotherapy, the classic line that comes up is: "Tell me about your mother." Psychiatry went as far as saying that schizophrenia is caused by a cold and insensitive mother. The term developed was a "schizophrenogenic mother" (meaning a mother that causes schizophrenia).

We now know that schizophrenia is a medical condition, and it is absurd to consider the fact that a mother could cause this by being "cold and distant." By the same token, it is very common for parents to be sensitive about being blamed for a child's struggles—particularly misbehavior.

Let's look at how parenting goes in most families. Parents have a child, and then they do the best they can at parenting. They may read one or many books, they may attend a parenting lecture or seminar through church or a local community center, and they learn some basic parenting principles. As their child grows up, the child presents different challenges based on different developmental stages. (Of course the issues of an eight year old are different than the issues of a three year old!)

Parents may reference other resources when they are challenged—which may even include asking their own parents—and then they make their best choice, and work out the issues. Most parents do not have to develop strict and structured parenting approaches, rather they adapt and follow basic principles, and things generally work out well. As their child grows up, these parents feel that their child has given them some challenges which were hard to handle (i.e. they gave them a "run for their money" at times), but that things worked out well. The parents are proud of themselves as parents, and they are proud of their child. This basic approach can be called **Natural Intuitive Parenting**.

In contrast to the parents described above, the parents of a child with ADD have their child, and begin in the same way. They read some books, or go to a lecture to learn some basic parenting principles. Yet—their son doesn't seem to respond to the approaches that everyone else describes. They quickly learn that when they use basic parenting principles and use their best judgement, it doesn't work with their child. This **Natural Intuitive Parenting** doesn't work with their ADD son or daughter.

The ADD parent then starts to put 10 times the effort into parenting compared to the parents of kids without ADD. And the results are often worse than what the other parents are getting. And to worsen the guilt and embarrassment of the parents of an ADD child, often times the behavior problems of their child can "blow up" in public. Then, the parent is mortified as others are looking at them with their out of control child—at the store, the park, the soccer game or at school. And the ADD parent knows that the other parents are judging them. And they feel shameful and embarrassed.

And the parents of non-ADD kids do judge. They think to themselves, "Just give me two days with that child, and I'll teach him how to behave. My child has done so well, under my guidance and support. That parent doesn't know what she's doing."

The reality is that the ADD parent puts 10 to 100 times more work into parenting than the other parents do, and the results are a lot less effective. The non-ADD parents have no concept of the severity of the challenges, yet they judge nonetheless.

So when the parent finally gets to the doctor, and gets a diagnosis of ADD for her son or daughter, there is some relief. There is now an explanation for the problems they've been having. And hope begins to shine a little light for these parents. And as the doctor discusses the treatment options for ADD, and gets to this section—i.e. parenting—the doctor suggests that the parents go for therapy—therapy which can happen without their child even needing to be there!

When the parent hears that she has to go for therapy, and that her child doesn't even have to attend, she feels blamed, upset and may lose any sense of hope that was developing. In fact, she can get angry at the doctor for saying this. She may feel that the doctor is confirming what her mother-in-law, neighbor or Aunt Sally said—that it's her fault.

This is where it is critically important to understand the role of parenting treatment in ADD, and how to approach it.

Parenting approaches in ADD can be summed up in one sentence:

Parents aren't the cause of ADD, but they can be part of the solution.

At the core of treatment for ADD is the implementation of structure. People with ADD struggle to set up their own internal structure, and they struggle to implement and maintain a structure if it is there. They need help to have structure around them. This likely relates to their struggles with executive functions—where they have trouble implementing structure in their own lives.

One of the issues with individual therapy—either cognitive, behavioral or insight oriented in children and teens with ADD—is that it is often not effective. This relates to the fact that kids and teens are often lacking the executive function of abstraction. This means taking the concept or learning from one environment and making the lesson abstract, and then applying that lesson to other situations. In other words, they have trouble generalizing a lesson from one environment to another.

I have witnessed kids who are taking part in a behavioral therapy for ADD; they do well in a therapy session which focused on helping them to stop and think before acting. In the session, they are following the steps recommended—stopping and thinking before acting. And then when their mom picks them up from the session, on the way to the elevator, they do something impulsive, and don't stop and think first. Did he forget the lesson? No. He still knows that when he is *in the therapy session*, he needs to follow those rules. But this is different; he is in the hallway near the elevator. He can learn the lesson, but he doesn't naturally generalize the lesson from the therapy session to outside of the therapy session—in all of the possible situations where it may come up—i.e. the hallway, the parking lot, school, home, the park, etc.

However, when the ADD child has a structure around him which helps him remember to implement strategies, then he is more likely to implement them, use them, and to do better in multiple areas of his life.

How can we make sure that there is structure around an ADD child, no matter where he or she goes?

The answer is—we have to teach it to the parents. Mom and dad have to set structure around their child, and make sure that the structure is implemented in multiple settings. Then, their child has a better chance to succeed.

Remember: Parents aren't the cause of ADD,
but they can be part of the solution.

This is why parenting strategies for ADD are a cornerstone for ADD treatment. Parents need to learn specialized techniques which will help their ADD child to function and to succeed. When they do, their child will start to do better in multiple settings—whether it is home, school, friend's houses, etc. And if parents are able to get some behavioral treatment for their child individually, then having had the parenting approaches in place will allow for those therapies to be more effective.

The need for parents to develop specific strategies to help with ADD is analogous to other medical conditions. For example, if a child has a peanut allergy, or diabetes, the parents need to learn about the condition, and they need to develop specific strategies to help their child. They also have to ensure that others will be able to help with their child when their child is in different settings. No parent is ashamed or feels guilty about having to learn how to help their newly diagnosed diabetic daughter—and it should be the same for ADD.

A Note about Family Makeup

When I discuss parents for kids and teens with ADD, I often refer to two parents, but I often use the pronoun *she*. That said, there is no research that shows that kids with ADD need two parents, one male and one female. Kids can do very well in single parent families, and they can do very well if they grow up with their grandparents, with two mommies, with foster families, etc.

The important thing is to pick up on the specific parenting principles and strategies, and implement them in your specific family makeup.

The Genetics of ADD

Remember that ADD often runs in families. That means that if one child has ADD, there is a chance that a second child has it, and there is also a chance that one (or both parents) have it as well.

When we are treating ADD, we are helping to set up a structure which is helpful. If the Mom (or Dad) has untreated ADD, then it could be very hard for her to set up a consistent structure for her son or daughter because it is hard to set up structures when there is untreated ADD.

If one parent has ADD traits, or actual ADD, it is important to talk to your own doctor about getting a diagnosis, and starting your own treatment. If you do, this can significantly improve your effectiveness as a parent. All of the strategies you use will be more effective, because it will be easier for you to use them consistently.

Core Principles and Strategies of Parenting for ADD

While there are many different systems for parenting for ADD, each of these systems has core underlying principles and strategies which must be in place for the system to work. As a child psychiatrist, I have reviewed many different parenting systems. I am including the most effective principles and strategies to help you with ADD. For many families, the material in this chapter will be enough to get you going in parenting effectively for ADD. For other families, you may want to review the approaches and get professional help with implementing a parenting approach that works well for your family.

The core principles and strategies for parenting include:

1. Building your parenting approach on a foundation of love
2. Consistency between parents
3. Knowing your parenting strengths
4. Knowing whoever is more flexible wins
5. Similar understanding of the cause of the symptoms
6. Implementing parenting approaches without anger
7. Choosing your battles
8. Letting go of the "Beaver Cleaver" archetype

9. Starting with a positive attitude

10. Developing the system, implementing and maintaining it

Let's begin to review these parenting principles and strategies:

1. BUILD YOUR PARENTING APPROACH ON A FOUNDATION OF LOVE

When you are working on your parenting approaches with your ADD child, it is critically important that you build upon a foundation of love.

As a parent myself, I know the power of a parent's love for his or her child. This is undeniable. As a psychiatrist, I frequently see that kids and teens don't believe that their parents love them because of the constant arguing, frustration and anger that they express. Or perhaps it's because the child feels that he continually lets mom down. It is very common for there to be a gap in understanding of the love that is actually there between the parent and the child.

How do you remind your child that you really do love them? How do you get them to feel it, and believe you?

Depending on the status of your relationship with your child or teen, you may have a little bit of work to do, or you may have a lot of work to do.

Irrespective of how much repair work you have to do, it all comes down to this: *You have to spend time with your child or teen, doing something they like, and showing your true interest in them and their life.*

When you are working on this, this is not the time to force them to take part in something that you want them to do that they have no interest in. Whether it is taking martial arts lessons, or going to church group—if you are imposing it, even though it may enrich your child's life in some way, it will not improve your loving bond, trust and communication with one another.

If you are in a situation where there is no clear answer—i.e. playing board games, or a multiplayer video game together (the Wii can be fun because the games are relatively simple and can be active), or something along those lines, then spend some time with your child asking what he'd like to do. Search for a passion of theirs that is not being met—maybe they want to play laser tag, or start art classes, or work on long distance bike riding. And then start it together. Put the time in, and be sure to not get into old patterns of communication where you just devolve into arguing about old issues. Make this a protected time so that you can enjoy one another and build your bond. Even though you know your child very well, if you do this right, you will learn a lot more about him or her.

While you are doing this—do your best to have simple yet meaningful moments. Times you do something silly or funny (especially if it is a mistake), laugh a lot about it—encourage your child to make fun of you over it. Laugh together and enjoy the fun together. Really, the fun, quiet and enjoyable moments are the ones that your child (and you!) need to establish and maintain the connection that is between you. The family bond, or blood connection is real, but you can be sure that it means a lot more to you than it does to your child. I have literally been talking with teens in my office who were trying to decide if their mother would care if they committed suicide—because she yelled at them on a daily basis. Your child or teen doesn't measure your relationship based on blood—he or she measures it based on the time you spend together, and the nature of that time together.

Spend more time with your child. Do fun things, and don't allow it to become about anger, discipline or frustrations. Consider this time as deposits in the **"bank of connection."** You need to keep a connection with your child so that he or she will listen to you, care about your opinion, and want to follow your requests. If you have no active connection with your child or teen, then they are much less likely to listen to you, or follow your advice.

Your child or teen has to *feel* that you love him or her.

How do you help them to feel this? You spend more time with them, let it be time about them, and listen to them. Don't just talk, or be directive. Let them do that. Be the supportive, loving parent that you are, and let them *experience* that, not just hear it from you. Aim to actually schedule your time with your child so that it happens at least weekly.

What should you do if your teen (or child) doesn't really talk to you about him or herself? You do everything right, and your teen doesn't talk. Be sure not to get upset with him or her. Specifically, be sure you don't say something like, "I'm trying to make a real effort here and you are contributing NOTHING. How can we improve our relationship if you don't care enough to even try?" This will shut your teen up even more, and make him or her resent the process even more.

If you are doing this right, and your teen isn't really talking—just talk about yourself. But make sure that you aren't talking about boring work issues, or about your belief in how your teen should improve his or her life. Talk about different things.

The best place to start is with your embarrassing moments. Yes—tell your teen about that time you spilled coffee all over yourself before the biggest meeting of your career; or how you really struck out when you were dating in high school; or how you really embarrassed yourself the first time you met your in-laws. Tell these funny stories, and laugh about them. Encourage your teen to enjoy your previous misfortunes. This type of discussion is not expected by your teen, and can help to change the nature of your communication (and possibly, relationship) for the better. This can be a starting point if the communication doesn't flow well right away.

2. CONSISTENCY BETWEEN PARENTS

When parents of a child *without* ADD work on parenting, they do not have to be perfectly consistent. Their child is "malleable" enough that if Mom has a slightly different approach than Dad, they aren't going to exploit that difference into bringing the family into chaos. However, an ADD child can routinely do that.

One of the core principles of parenting an ADD child is that there has to be complete consistency. If the child knows that if he just persists longer, Mom will cave in, then he will persist longer. If he knows that certain requests get Dad to say yes, even if Mom will say no, he will wait until he can ask Dad.

And if there is some difference between Mom and Dad's response, and (even better from the child's perspective) they argue about it—the child will exploit this so that Mom and Dad break out into an argument, and then the child can either get what he or she wants, or he can make Mom and Dad suffer for not granting it to him. When Mom and Dad start arguing, it deflects the attention from the child, and onto Mom and Dad's relationship or parenting, and the child "wins."

For any parenting approach to be successful with an ADD child, it has to be "bullet proof"—i.e. completely consistent. If it isn't, the child will find the "wiggle room," and exploit it for his benefit.

How Do Parents Develop Consistency?

Consistency can be a challenge to develop, for several reasons. Firstly, as mentioned above, if either Mom or Dad has ADD, it can be hard to be consistent, without treatment and insight into that condition.

Secondly, Mom and Dad likely had different experiences with their own parents when they were growing up. Maybe Dad's parents were strict and forced obedience, whereas Mom's parents talked things through to get to the "emotional meanings" behind issues. Or even worse, maybe one set of parents were physically or emotionally abusive. If the parents of an ADD child come from such different backgrounds, then it could be hard for them to agree on an approach for their own child—especially if the stress level is climbing for them in their family.

And the parents' own experience with their parents is very relevant to how they parent. Many people say that they will never do the same things that their parents did to them. Whether they do or don't, their own parents set a "template" which has a great influence on how they parent. Many parents are surprised when they hear words coming out of their own mouth which are words that they hated hearing from their own parents when they were young. Most people end up taking on a similar parenting style to their own mother or father. Or, they do the exact opposite.

Understanding the strong influence of your own parents on your parenting style can make a big difference in helping you to choose the best parenting approach that suits your family now—rather than just "running old patterns" which you got from your family of origin. It can also help to explain why some of the things that your spouse (or co-parent) does drives you crazy.

Working on this aspect of consistency can be done quite effectively with a therapist, if you are struggling with it on your own.

Defining Clear Expectations and Goals

If I took you to an archery range, blindfolded you, spun you around, and then told you to shoot at the target, how would you do? Probably not well (and I'd be ducking!).

If you don't know what your target is, it's hard to hit it.

Yet, most parents are trying to implement rules and goals which are not defined, and are unclear. And worse yet, they may be slightly different depending on whether it is Mom or Dad who is articulating them in the moment.

Parents need to set clear expectations, goals and rules.

This means sitting down, brainstorming, writing down, and agreeing on what they are going to be. Then, writing them out briefly, concisely, and posting them somewhere obvious (like in the kitchen, or hallway upstairs for more privacy). When they are posted, you go over them with your child or teen.

There is something powerful about expectations, goals and rules which are written down. It is not longer dependent on whether Mom is there or Dad is there, or whether they are tired, stressed out, or too busy to spend time on this right now. The rules are the rules. And they are posted.

When the rules are posted, it is hard for your child or teen to "wiggle" around them.

Aim for this as a goal to improve your parenting.

Role Playing

One of the tasks of being consistent with rules and expectations is to consider all of the ways that things may go wrong. When you consider all of the different angles that your son or daughter will use to defy these rules, you can figure out the best way(s) to handle it.

This is where you can "role play" handling discipline moments to practice the best approaches. One parent can play the role of the child (you know what he or she says when being defiant), and the other parent can practice handling the situation. If you are a single parent, you can do this with a friend, a therapist, or you can even write it out in a journal to practice your response. Get good at clearly enforcing the rules and expectations, and implementing the consequences. Refer to your written rules.

These steps will help you to be consistent between parents—which is crucial to successfully parenting an ADD child or teen.

3. KNOW YOUR PARENTING STRENGTHS

The third core principle of ADD is that each parent has to know his/her strengths and weaknesses as a parent.

If there are two parents in your family, you are no doubt aware that one parent has the ability to handle certain circumstances better than the other. To put it another way, it is pretty clear that one parent always struggles when in a particular situation. For example, maybe dad doesn't have the patience to help with homework, but he is great for bedtime. Or maybe mom loses her cool with getting him out the door in the morning, but dad does it really well. If you are able to acknowledge what your strengths are, and what the strengths are of your co-parent, then you can split tasks based on these, to the best of your abilities.

If you are a single parent, this is still very important. Granted, most of the tasks will fall to you, but if you can identify the tasks you do very well—i.e. your strengths, and you can identify your weaknesses, you can then develop specific strategies to help you to function better. For example, if you struggle with homework time, you may be able to get a tutor, or an after school program where your child gets her homework done. And if finances are a challenge to pay for it, see if you can find a senior student who needs to get her volunteer hours, or a student from your church who would be willing to help. Some creativity may help you to get the support you need.

4. WHOEVER IS MORE FLEXIBLE WINS

Let's imagine the classic situation of a parent and child nearing the grocery store checkout. The child sees the ten dollar toy that is put near the cash register, and starts asking (or whining?) for this toy. As the parent, you don't want to get them the toy, because it's a waste of money, and you know that your child will play with it for five minutes, and then never touch it again (at least not after they leave it on the stairs for someone to trip on…). When you say no, your child starts a scene. Whether it is crying, moaning, threatening, or a full blown temper tantrum, they start and don't want to stop. And then the parent tries to say no in several ways until they give up, just to end the terribly embarrassing display of behavior.

When this type of situation happens, there is a clear mathematical formula for this: **Whoever is more flexible, wins.** If the son has 25 ways to demand the toy, and the mom has four ways to say no, then the son is always going to win. Especially because he will escalate his ways to request the toy in order to push mom's emotional buttons. If he knows that mom gets embarrassed when he cries—he'll cry, as soon as he thinks that mom is seriously refusing the request. If crying doesn't work for some reason (i.e. mom is strengthening her resolve), then he'll try several other behaviors to see which will work, possibly learning a new emotional hot button to reuse on mom on another day.

If this type of pattern develops, your son or daughter is essentially doing behavioral field research on you, running multiple emotional and behavioral experiments on you to find your hot buttons, to reuse when they really want something on another day.

How do you stop this version of torture that your child is trying to inflict on you? Whether it's in the grocery store, or some other embarrassing situation?

You need to develop more flexibility than your child. For most parents, that means letting go of your embarrassment. Embarrassment is often the key that leads to parents losing these types of battles. When you get embarrassed as a parent, you are willing to give in, because it is just too hard to stick with your resolve and keep your point.

When you let go of the possibility of you becoming embarrassed in these types of circumstances, you open the door for you to maintain your position as the parent, and win that particular battle.

In this type of general discussion, I can't tell you exactly what you can do for your particular circumstance. Spend some time brainstorming what you can do which is more flexible than your child. Maybe your child hates when you sing Michael Jackson—because your voice is terrible, and when you shake your hips, it's totally embarrassing. If this is the case, make it clear to your son that after you've asked three times, you will stop what you're doing until you get the chorus of *Thriller* done.

A colleague of mine—a family therapist—has teenagers, and they play on various sports teams. When he asks them to leave, or follow rules, they can become challenging at times. They have made it clear that it is totally embarrassing to them when he takes off his shirt. If they don't listen to his reasonable requests after a game, he'll let them know that he's feeling hot and wants to take off his shirt, and then they will comply.

Now, you may think that it's bizarre for a child psychiatrist to tell you to do something absurd to have your child change his or her behavior. But this child psychiatrist is telling you just that. You don't have to necessarily embarrass yourself, but what you do need to do is to be willing to prove to your child that you are willing to do whatever it takes—you are willing to be more flexible than he is to stick to your point. And that you are willing to experiment over and over until you find a way that works.

As an aside, kids develop tremendous persistence when it comes to life. When they are learning to walk, they don't try once or twice, say that it doesn't work, and give up. They keep trying until they succeed. And if they want the new video game for the computer, they don't ask once or twice and give up—they keep trying, in various different ways, to see if they can get Mom or Dad to give in. Yet, there are many parents that I see who try one, or two, or even three ways to help to maintain the discipline with their child, and then they give up. They say, "I tried that system and it doesn't work, Nothing can help my child." And while I acknowledge that it can be tremendously frustrating and challenging, most parents don't realize that they are often just a few steps from success when they give up.

Before kids and teens will "say uncle" and give in to your new rules, they will put up the strongest resistance ever. The first time you try to implement your new rule or approach, your child will fight hardest. They are testing your resolve to see if you are serious—whether you mean business. If you can maintain your position, your child will fight less hard on the second time around, even less by the third, and then he or she will settle in to the new order. This is only true *if* you maintain consistency. If you show a lack of consistency, your child will fight harder each time, to see if they can break your resolve each time.

When it comes to some parent's concerns regarding the willingness to do something which could be embarrassing to themselves in order to help their child, I think of two things:

Firstly, I think of a wonderful family that I work with who has a son with severe autism. He is non-verbal, and he can run away at times with no warning. Now that he's more than 10 years old, he can be very fast when he runs. His father was telling me that when they have gone to hotels to take part in conventions/meetings for autism—his son has taken off from the shower—completely naked. And Dad, often naked as well, had to run after his son to ensure his safety—immediately. I'm not sure what *you* may be embarrassed about, but I can be pretty sure that it isn't as bad as it was for that Dad.

Secondly, I think of wise words that a friend shared with me, and I'll paraphrase them here: Do what you need to do to parent. Because those who mind don't matter, and those who matter don't mind!

The bottom line here? Work on your flexibility, and be willing to try many different ways to help your child and to impose the proper rules and discipline on him or her. If you read this section and feel that you are not resourceful enough in this moment to find the "right way" to approach this with your child, talk to your child's doctor or therapist and see if you can develop some approaches which will work.

5. SIMILAR UNDERSTANDING OF THE CAUSE OF THE SYMPTOMS

As a practicing child psychiatrist, I see many kids and teens with their parents. Most often, one parent comes into the office with the child for their follow-up visits, and that is most commonly the mother (sometimes it is the Dad, though not that frequently).

When I get the opportunity to visit with both parents (which can be important at times for a particular family), I will often ask the parents if they agree on the nature of their child's symptoms, and what is causing them. And then I am often amazed by what I hear.

Even if both parents are quite educated (University/College), there is often one parent who has read more on the condition, attended more appointments, and had more discussions with professionals. As previously mentioned, this is often the mother. The mother is therefore often the expert on the condition in the family. When I ask the mother if she understands the cause of her son's symptoms, she often gives a good explanation of how the ADD impacts her son and causes the symptoms and/or behaviors. However, the less involved parent (often the Dad), generally starts out with "saying the right things." Though when pushed a little further, the second parent often will share some misconceptions about his child's behavior. Things like: "I know he's capable, and I think he just doesn't want to try." Or, even more concerning, "I think he'd do fine if his mother didn't indulge him so much."

If one parent has an underlying belief that undermines the first parent, then this causes significant problems, and makes it hard for any specific strategies to work. Even if the child doesn't hear daddy say these things to mommy, he knows that Dad is blaming Mom, and there is inconsistency for him to exploit.

It is really important for both parents to gain the same understanding of what causes the symptoms, and support one another with it. This means agreeing strongly enough so that when a mother-in-law, or a concerned aunt shares a news story about how ADD isn't real—how it is only caused by pesticides (or some other fashionable news story of the month). Then both parents will be able to correct that misconception, support the other parent, and justify the reasons and needs for the treatments and approaches required for their child.

Realize this—the parents would certainly do that for a diabetic child if someone got in the way of their child's treatment plan, diagnosis, or the need to follow certain approaches to maintain his or her health.

6. IMPLEMENT PARENTING APPROACHES WITHOUT ANGER

One of the most important things about implementing discipline with your child is that you need to implement the discipline *without anger, guilt or shame.*

Think about how society upholds laws in your neighborhood. If you are driving in a 15 mph zone, and you are doing 30 mph, and the police officer pulls you over, how does the conversation go? It's something along these lines:

Police Officer: "License and registration please. Do you know how fast you were going?"

Motorist: "I'm sorry officer, I'm late for work."

Police Officer: "Well, you were going 30 mph, and you broke the speed limit. Here is your ticket. Remember, this is a school zone."

Realize that the police officer handles this situation professionally, and clearly. Here are the elements of this interaction about breaking a rule:

- There is a rule which is posted (15 mph).

- The police officer clearly explains how the rule was broken, and gives out the consequence. The consequence is given right away, and the officer doesn't wait until a time at some point in the future to give you punishment.

- The consequence is clear, and you know what it is even before you get your ticket (i.e. you know you will get demerit points, and a fine).

- The police officer doesn't make up the consequence in the moment, and the consequence wouldn't be different based on which officer is present at the scene.

- The police officer does not yell at you, doesn't degrade you, and doesn't bring up all of the things that you've done wrong in the past.

- The police officer doesn't take 30 minutes to explain the reason why speed limits are in place, and engage in the ensuing "intellectual debate" about the merits of speed limits and whether they should even exist.

- If you refuse to accept the ticket, or get too angry at the officer, or even if you get aggressive with the officer, there are clear consequences as to what will happen (most likely, it will be escalated quickly, and you will get arrested for assaulting a police officer).

When it comes to disciplining your child, be like this police officer. As you can plainly see, there are key elements to handling discipline:

1. Have a clear rule which is posted.

2. Have a clear consequence if the rule is broken.

3. Have clear consequences for bad behavior which comes as a result of the discipline (i.e. excessive anger, swearing, aggression).

4. Have a clear, BRIEF, discussion when a rule is broken, and give the known consequence clearly at the time of the incident.

5. Follow through on the consequence, and ensure it is done as written.

In element four above, I have capitalized the word "brief." This is where most parents fall down. We live in a talking society. We feel that we have to explain ourselves to our children. And we believe that if we could only explain it the right way, our child will finally understand.

If I had a nickel for each time a mother says to her son that he shouldn't hit his sister, thinking that if she explains it better this time, he may finally get it. When parents do this, they are making the assumption that their child is just missing the right information to make the best choice. In other words, if the brother finally realized that it actually hurt his sister when he hit her, he would say, "Oh my gosh. Thank you for explaining that. Now that I get it, I will never do that again!"

Of course this doesn't happen, because the son already knows that it is wrong to hit his sister, but he can't control himself in the moment that he gets angry. When this happens, he needs to understand the consequence—but without a big explanation (just like the example with the police officer).

When parents get into a long explanation about the rules or the consequences, the child starts to argue or negotiate the issue. What results is not productive. The child aggravates the parent, starts to build his/her own resolve, and at the end of the day, the rule still has to apply. Remember how there is no way that the police officer is going to get into a philosophical debate about whether speeding tickets should even exist?

One other trap that parents walk into is bringing up past issues. If there is a problem from today, mom brings up the incident from last Thursday, and the week before that, as well as the thing that happened at grandma's three months ago. This most likely is to happen during this heated argument about the rules—which shouldn't even be happening. When a parent brings up all of the old offences, it takes this discipline moment out of the present moment—the now—and creates multiple emotional issues which cause anger, frustration and more misbehavior. Keep things simple—just focus on the issue of today, and get it resolved appropriately. When you do this regularly, you won't have to bring up old issues—because the issue from last Thursday will have been dealt with last Thursday.

Be a police officer. Enforce the rule. Don't get into a discussion about it.

Knowing what I know from my office, there is a high percentage of parents who will insist: "but I have to explain things to my child. I can't just not talk to him."

The answer to this is clear:

- During a discipline moment, don't say any more than the bare minimum to make the point and enforce the discipline. Some parents have to walk away to stop themselves from over explaining and ruining the discipline.

- When it is not a discipline moment, talk to your son or daughter as much as possible. Talk about why the sky is blue and clouds look white. Talk about how the internet works, and how you didn't have computers when you were young, etc.

When it is not a discipline moment, should you talk about the rules and expectations? This can be quite appropriate if it is done in the correct way. For example, you could have a discussion with your child about the appropriate punishment (i.e., A or B) if he breaks the rule, but you can't have a discussion about the fact that the rule shouldn't exist. In this same way, a citizen of a democracy, with its rules, could choose to get involved in the political process to provide input into the proper punishments for perpetrators of crime.

The most important point is this: if you get angry when you are trying to discipline your child, you make the whole issue shift to an emotional one, and your child will react to your anger. Most of the time, your child will get emotionally upset, and will draw incorrect conclusions about how you feel about them based on your anger (i.e. you don't love me because you yelled). They take the lesson that "mommy doesn't love me," instead of "if I hit my sister, I lose my privileges and have to go to my room." And in many circumstances, if your child feels that you aren't giving him or her enough time, they may act out to get some active emotions out of you—i.e. anger is better than nothing.

The bottom line? Do enough preparation work, so that you know what the consequences are going to be, and so does your child. If he or she breaks the rules, act like you are a police officer, just enforcing the law. No anger or drama necessary. Don't get into long discussions. Don't bring up previous "offences." Just keep it simple and to the point. And after the "discipline moment" is over, take some time to be with your child—playing, doing an activity, or something together. You need to have a relationship beyond the discipline.

7. CHOOSE YOUR BATTLES

Many families get quite upset over many issues with their ADD children. No matter what happens, she never seems to remember to hang up her jacket on the hook when she comes into the house. You think to yourself: "It's so simple—why can't she just do it?" and, "If I ever threw my jacket on the ground when I was a kid like she does, my parents would have given me the belt (or some other awful punishment)."

My advice to you for these smaller issues which lead to day-to-day arguing?

Let them go.

Pick the important things, focus your efforts there, and accept that her jacket may be on the ground for 300+ days per year.

This message is very important for parents of teenagers. I frequently hear of messy rooms and the battles over them. I hear about how the teen won't talk to Mom about anything, but all Mom wants to talk about is the messy room, and some other things around the house that should be done. This leads to frequent anger on both sides of the relationship, and often this leads to complete communication breakdown between the parent and the teen.

This is where parents are not serving themselves or their teens. During the teen years, most teens in Western society will be faced with decisions which will have major impacts on their futures, and their current safety. Things like: driving, alcohol, drugs and sex. These so-called "activities" can lead to teen death (motor vehicle accidents are a leading cause of death in teens), teen pregnancy, criminal behavior, addiction, school dropout, etc.

Parents want to teach the proper values and beliefs to their teens, yet they can't have a civil, five minute conversation with them because they've been fighting over things like: the laundry on their bedroom floor, leaving their jacket open during the winter, or not eating supper at the same time as everyone else.

As a parent, you need to allow for natural consequences.

You need to allow your teen to screw up, and then let life teach them a lesson. And you need to be there to support them if you can.

Rather than yell at your daughter every cold day for four years about doing up her jacket in the cold weather so she won't catch pneumonia, let her go out as she wants. If she does catch pneumonia, just be reassured that we have a good healthcare system, and she can get treatment. She will learn that she needs to zip up in cold weather, and then you won't have to fight about it.

And if you can let go of the winter jacket issue (and all of these more "minor" issues), there is a better chance that you will be able to discuss with your daughter how to handle it when people offer her marijuana, or how to practice abstinence or safe sex. In other words, if you drive your teen crazy over day-to-day stuff, then you have no opportunity to be involved in the important things. If you stay out of it, you can let life teach your teen lessons and you may be able to be involved in the more important issues.

Some parents reading this will think that I am suggesting that you give up any standards for your child. This is just not the case.

I suggest that you allow your child to experience "natural consequences" around issues which are not that important in the grand scheme of things.

For example, if your teen is late for school, let the school administration deal with her rather than having a major battle each morning. If your teen doesn't get school work done, let the teacher give the consequences for not completing work. If your teen leaves her clothes on the bedroom floor, close the door, and let her wear wrinkled, dirty clothes to school. At some point, she is going to get embarrassed and want to wear something clean and fresh smelling. There are worse things in this world than having your teen wear dirty clothes...

The bottom line is that you have to choose the battles that are important to win. Let go of some of the things that seem important, though really aren't.

8. LET GO OF THE "BEAVER CLEAVER" ARCHETYPE

Our society is full of archetypes that many families try to live up to. One of them is the "Beaver Cleaver" family—the family from the 50s TV series *Leave it to Beaver*. In this archetypal family, there is a professional Dad, a stay at home Mom, and the "right moral code" for an American family. Even though many parents don't say that they aspire to this type of archetype, often unconsciously, that is exactly what they are doing.

Many families have thoughts about how things are supposed to be. For example, many families believe that a child has to sit quietly and politely during the supper/dinner meal, so that all of the family members can be together, and discuss their day. If this is important to your family, you no doubt find it frustrating, if not infuriating when your ADD son takes two bites, gets up from the table and runs around, to return three minutes later to take two more bites.

This point ties in nicely with the last point of "choosing your battles." You need to decide if having a "family dinner" in the way that you used to have it, or would like to have it is realistic for your family. It may not be, and you may need to let it go.

Rather than rely on the archetypal ideas—like a family supper time, why not find something that suits your family, and the unique nature of each individual? Maybe it is an after supper activity—like a walk or a bike ride—that each can participate in.

Or maybe it is not doing something as a family.

You may have to "divide and conquer."

In many families with ADD, it can be too hard to have all of the family members spend time together. There can be battles, fights, or challenges. And what is intended to bring the family together can lead to people growing further apart.

The concept of "family togetherness" is a noble one, though it is not written in stone, and it is not necessary. It comes from one of those Beaver Cleaver archetypes. Depending on the nature of your family, you may do better to split your kids up between parents (or if you're a single parent, you may need to split with grandparents and/or a friend) to do different activities. And that way, each child can have their needs met, without the terrible battles.

The bottom line is this: rather than hold your family to an archetype that may not actually suit your family, be realistic about who your family members are, what their strengths and weaknesses are, and make the best choices you can about how to live your lives together in the way that is best for all of you. This may mean breaking down some of the archetypes or stereotypes that you are carrying around in your mind (sometimes without even realizing it). The best way to become aware of some of these unconscious stereotypes is to think about the things that you want to have happen in your family, and things that make you the angriest when they don't happen. That emotional reaction gives you the clue to the fact that that issue is a great place to start.

9. START WITH POSITIVITY

When developing a "discipline system," it is very important to start with positivity.

When your child is doing something that is a negative behavior, you want him to stop the negative behavior, and replace it with a positive behavior as an alternative. Most of the time, you'll get better results if you start to encourage the positive behavior first, and then punish the negative behavior later.

If your child has been struggling with not listening to the soccer coach, and disrupting the soccer games, then the positive behavior in this case which you want to promote is to listen to the soccer coach. Before you start to punish your child for not listening, I encourage you to develop a reward system for showing the good behavior of listening to the coach. The reward can be stickers, or "points" which are collected and redeemed later on for a small reward. Promote the positive behavior effectively, and you may not have to punish the negative behavior at all.

When it comes to setting up a reward system, it is important to keep it simple—and appropriate to your child's age. Make the tasks which are rewarded clear, and don't make the list too long. Set up a chart, which is displayed prominently—maybe on the fridge for all to see. If you can choose three to five things as tasks to reward, this is a great place to start. Be clear on how these will be monitored, and how the rewards will be reviewed. It is best to do this more frequently (i.e. at least daily)—because if your child feels like he's being good and you're not even noticing, or forgetting to reward him, he'll give up on the system. Whereas if he can see daily progress, he will be propelled to keep going.

When it comes to rewards, there should be some system for your child to trade in his points or stickers for something good. Many parents make the mistake of making this a huge item that takes a long time to get. For example, it is far better to have frequent rewards with small knick-knacks from the dollar store, than to make your child save up points for four months to win a video game console. If the reward is too far ahead, and seems unattainable, then your child will have trouble sticking to the system.

Also, don't set the reward as a family trip. I have had many parents who encourage their child to get the reward of a trip to a theme park (i.e. a family trip to Disneyworld), and then they struggle when the tickets are bought and their son is now misbehaving and not following the system. What kind of message does it give their child if he gets the reward when he didn't do the work to get it? But it's also hard to cancel a trip that's paid for because your son didn't earn enough tokens (try telling that to the travel agent or travel insurance agent). It's best to keep the rewards to smaller items which are rewarded more frequently.

Once your child begins to follow the reward system, and succeed with it, begin to include punishment or consequence for the negative behavior that must be avoided. This approach helps your child get the positivity first— i.e. feeling good about doing well, and then suffer the consequences later on if he doesn't follow through as he should.

10. DEVELOP THE SYSTEM, IMPLEMENT AND MAINTAIN

When you are working on parenting for an ADD child or teen, you need to put a lot of work up front into setting up the right approach. You need to reference different resources (like this book), as well as therapists, doctors, or other community resources to set up a system that is right for you and your family. Your child will likely show resistance to the changes you are going to make, and you may resist some of the ideas that you'll actually need to accept to make progress. Get help to develop the right system for you.

Once you have the right system in place, you will need to implement it. Remember, when you first implement the system, you will get the most resistance from your child at that point. It will be the hardest for you in the beginning. You need to set up some support for yourself when you first implement, so that you can stick to it, and make it work.

And once it is going, you'll need to work on maintaining this system. You'll need to adapt as new issues come up. You'll need to adapt as your child gets older, and reaches successively, different developmental stages. And you'll have to watch yourself, so that when things get better, you don't "loosen up" on your rules and expectations, which can undo all of your hard work.

Parenting a child or teen with ADD can be a tremendous challenge, and it can also be tremendously rewarding when you are successful.

Other Resources

There are many helpful resources out there to help parents with their ADD kids and teens. If you would like to read more, I recommend the following resources:

1. *Taking Charge of ADHD*   By Dr. Russell Barkley

2. *1,2,3 Magic*   By Dr. Thomas Phelan

3. *Surviving Your Adolescents*   By Dr. Thomas Phelan

These books provide approaches and concepts similar to those presented here, and may help you further.

If you are struggling with significant explosive behavior, or defiance which is completely out of control, then I suggest you consider *The Explosive Child* by Dr. Ross Greene.

In this book, Dr. Greene shares a different approach for children who may have ADD or other disorders like autism, bipolar, etc., who are displaying significant lack of flexibility, and significant explosive behavior.

CHAPTER 6

Step 4: School and Academic Strategies for ADD

O nce a diagnosis is made, and you implement parenting strategies, it is important to develop strategies which are going to help your child or teen in school. It is very common that school issues are the main reason that people are referred for assessment of ADD. The teacher notes that your son or daughter is struggling in school. He's distractible, he's not getting his work done, and he's not achieving his potential.

When it comes to you (as a parent) helping your child or teen with school, the core foundation of achieving this is good communication between the parent(s) and the teacher(s), as well as the school administration. This is not always easy, and it can depend a lot on the individuals involved.

In my experience, there are often big differences between how one school handles kids with ADD compared to another—even when they are in the same school board. It often has to do with the individual's experience with ADD—whether it is the principal, vice-principal, guidance counsellor, or teacher. In general, if the school staff has personal experience with ADD, they tend to help a lot more. They do this because they know that with just a little extra effort on their part, your child can do a lot better. There are also school personnel who just don't "get it," and they say things like: "Now that he's in sixth grade, we shouldn't have to spoon feed him; that just isn't going to prepare him for 7th grade." They are missing the core understanding of the challenges with ADD, and how the changes (which are often minor) can make dramatic differences for the student with ADD.

And then there are times that teachers have a completely ignorant understanding of ADD. A teen recently told me that his 9th grade teacher told him that getting an A on one test was the worst thing that he could have done. The teacher said: "Now that I know you're capable of getting an A, that proves that you aren't trying the rest of the time." This angered the teen, de-motivated him, and made him feel completely misunderstood. The reality is that when people have "Attention Difference Disorder," they pay attention differently. They may have moments of brilliance, or great results, followed by days or weeks of struggles. It's that inconsistency or difference that is the hallmark of ADD, rather than a persistent "deficit." This teacher lacked that understanding and instead held a good test result against this student and made him feel that it just isn't worth putting forth good efforts.

Of course, when we can get teachers and school administrators to really understand the nature of ADD and take a strength-based approach to ADD, then it can be tremendous for your child (as well as the other students who come to the school after your child ...). As we discussed in Chapter 2, the "Parent's ADD Journey" means that parents go from being students to experts to advocates. When parents take the opportunity to educate their own child's school about ADD and their child's particular needs, this is one of the best places to begin advocacy. And it can have a very high yield for your child in so far as benefits and outcomes.

Sometimes the relationship with the school and the parents doesn't get off on the "right foot." This can relate to the fact that often it is the teacher or school administration who suggest that the parents should take their child to the doctor to get an assessment for ADD. This is completely appropriate for teachers to say, if they are seeing some issues of concern.

Unfortunately, sometimes teachers go too far in their suggestions. They say something like: "Your child has ADD. Get him to the doctor and on some medicine, or I just won't be able to keep him in my class." In my experience, it is relatively rare that a teacher makes this kind of statement in this day and age, but it still does happen. The teacher's comment above is wrong in a few ways:

1) Teachers can't diagnose a medical condition. So even if they suspect ADD, they can only suggest you go and see your doctor for an assessment.

2) Teachers can't recommend treatment. Teachers can't assess whether medication is needed for your child, and they certainly can't prescribe it.

3) Teachers can't demand a medical treatment in order for your child to receive an education, i.e., "if your son isn't on Ritalin®, I won't be able to keep him in this class."

Although it's very rare (in my experience) that teachers start out in this way, when they do, it sets a negative tone for the parents to work with the teachers. Fortunately, it seems to be occurring less frequently in recent years than it used to. If a teacher does start off with you in this way, be sure to speak to the teacher and/or school administration about the fact that you intend to take your child for an assessment, but you feel uncomfortable with the nature of the teacher's diagnosis and treatment recommendations, and that you would prefer to listen to the doctor's assessment and recommendations.

Even if the teacher is being unreasonable, and even if the school administration is not being helpful—it is ultimately your responsibility to advocate for your child, and nurture a good working relationship with the school. Even if you are "right," but if the school is making things miserable for your child, your child isn't going to succeed.

Sometimes parents can get very defensive about their children and how the school is handling it. And although the parents may be right, being defensive doesn't help to find solutions to get your child started learning and succeeding in school. If anything, it leads to more frustration and clashes with the school administration. So, it is best to get resourceful; work with your doctor and therapists to find solutions which will work, and do your best to cooperate with the school.

In most cases, when a teacher suggests an assessment for ADD, it is based on their view that your child is experiencing a higher than expected level of inattention, hyperactivity or impulsivity based on their age and stage of development. This can be very helpful information, and a great way to start the process of assessment and treatment. Most of the time, the teacher's insight helps you to get things on track for your child or teen, and thus the teacher is doing you a great service by informing you of his/her concerns.

If you do end up in the position that a teacher really doesn't "get" your child, it can be a hard year. Once you realize that you can't get things to change for this year, do your best to have input and to provide advice regarding which teacher your son or daughter will get next year.

One of the aspects of a kid's academic performance is that the teacher can have a big impact on how well your son or daughter does academically in any given year. Kids and teens with ADD will do really well with a teacher who's engaging, animated, and sees their gifts within them; whereas they may do a lot worse if they have a teacher who operates "by-the-book" and doesn't think they should have to spoon-feed anybody or treat anybody differently. When that happens, the ADD child or teen can feel misunderstood, become defiant and "turn" on the teacher.

Things can get a lot worse. If you can maintain a good working relationship with the school, and have some input into whom your child's teacher is for the next academic year, that can make a big difference to your child's performance over time.

In summary, the first key to your child succeeding at school is good communication between you and the school. Work hard at this, as it can yield great results.

Getting Official Support In School

In the U.S., kids and teens can actually get official recognition for ADD and get academic support. This official recognition is not present in other countries. That said, even in systems where there's no official recognition for ADD, people can still get some extra help or support with good advocacy and good energy put into it. In the US, parents can refer to the IDEA and 504 legislation to get help for their child or teen.

Children or teens with ADD may be eligible under the IDEA—the Individuals with Disabilities Education Act. This applies when the ADD is determined to be: "A chronic or acute health problem which adversely affects educational performance." This is often the case with ADD. When this legislation is used, the ADD individual is classified as OHI—other health impaired—and the school must develop an IEP (Individual Educational Plan) to meet your son or daughter's educational needs.

The 504 legislation refers to Section 504 of the Rehabilitation Act of 1973. It is a law that prevents any kind of discrimination in any program which receives federal funding to run—including education. It provides for access to a free and *appropriate* public education for all children, regardless of their disability. It states that children with disabilities need to be provided with the same opportunities that children without disabilities receive. To qualify under section 504, the student must:

- Be determined to have a physical or mental disability which substantially limits one or more major life activity, including learning and behaviour,
- Have a record of this impairment, and
- Be regarded as having such impairment.

If your child is determined to meet the criteria for 504, the school will make sure that he or she has "equal access to education." The school will then create accommodations or modifications tailored to his/her individual needs.

Outside of the US, there is generally less official recognition for ADD in the school systems. In Ontario, Canada, where I work, there is no official recognition for ADD in the school system. Children can get "identified" for requiring special support if they meet criteria for a learning disability (with or without ADD), an emotional or behavioral problem, or other possible criteria as established by the school board. In Ontario, the criteria are established by the Ministry of Education. If a child just has ADD, he will not receive official support within the school.

Although school boards may vary in different regions, a basic structure of how schools work with respect to kids who are experiencing difficulties is outlined below.

A Basic Structure

The school has a committee which meets regularly (usually monthly) so that school staff (specifically teachers and administrators) can discuss any child who is experiencing difficulties. The student could be struggling for any reason at all, including parental divorce, illness in the family, or ADD. In the Toronto District School Board, this is called the ISST, which stands for the *In School Support Team*. The ISST will review the student's current issues and challenges, and decide if any steps are needed to help the student. If it is necessary, they will refer the child to the next step in the process.

The next step is a committee called the SST, which stands for the *School Support Team*. The SST includes the school staff—i.e. teachers and administrators—and the SST also includes other professionals who can get involved to help out. This includes school psychologists, social workers, and speech and language therapists. Before this meeting happens, parents are sent a letter to let them know that their child is being brought forward for discussion in this meeting. Parents can actually refuse to have their child discussed at this meeting, though the school would try to educate the parent about the fact that this will be quite helpful in identifying the student's strengths and weaknesses (which are often referred to as "needs" or "challenges"). The SST can decide if the student needs further assessment—i.e. psychological testing, speech and language assessment, or an assessment with the school social worker. If testing is suggested, once the testing is completed, the results are brought back to the SST for review and to determine which remedies can be helpful. The SST has the ability to provide some support to the student—including actually creating an IEP—an Individual Educational Plan.

If there is a need for specific identification of the student's difficulties, the student is referred to the *Identification, Placement and Review Committee*, or IPRC. The IPRC's goal is to identify students as "exceptional," and to deem which help and resources can be helpful to them. Students can be deemed exceptional for any of a number of reasons, including:

- Being gifted intellectually,
- Having learning disabilities,
- Having an emotional problem,
- Having a behaviour problem,
- Mild Intellectual Disability/Developmental Disability,
- Having a physical disability,
- Etc.

Please remember that your school board may have different criteria for recognizing a student as exceptional. As mentioned previously, in the US, ADD can lead to a student meeting criteria for identification and support, whereas in most other places, it doesn't.

The IPRC is comprised of three objective school personnel—including a principal (who doesn't know the student), a psychologist (who didn't test and doesn't know the student) and a special education teacher (who doesn't know the student). The goal is that this committee will look at the testing results, the student's strengths and weaknesses, and not be biased by personal interactions with the student. The parent is invited to attend the IPRC, and the parent is also able to bring along others to the meeting, such as a doctor, a psychologist, or even an educational advocate. The parent does have the right to refuse to have his child reviewed at the IPRC. I generally advise against this course of action, as it blocks the school from providing the support that is needed for your child.

Parents can request an IPRC at any time even if there has not been any assessment done and the school board is obligated to provide one.

Once the IPRC reviews the testing data and information gathered about the student, they will decide if the student meets criteria for exceptionality. If the student does, the IPRC will create an IEP.

The IEP (Individual Education Plan) is a legal document which is a work in progress. This means that it requires ongoing review and updating. The IEP summarizes the strengths and weaknesses of the student, and the support needed. It contains a column to document what level the student is working at, a column for what they are working on (and the support provided), and then a column for when they have achieved that goal. Then, the next step is begun, and as such, the IEP is a continually evolving document, or a work in progress.

The IPRC committee decides which accommodations and modifications can be helpful for your child. They can recommend that your child is placed in a different classroom. The options can include:

- Regular class.

- Regular class with support—this would include withdrawal by a special education teacher or other professional from the regular class as deemed necessary.

- Special education class, at the home school program—this includes being in a separate class in the home school. There can be integration for some of the courses which are not areas of concern.

- Special education class intensive support program. This is usually a regional program, meaning that there is one school per area that has this program, and your child may have to move to a different school. The students spend most of the day in this self- contained class with integration as tolerated, usually for classes like gym, music, or art. These classes are either just Learning Disability classes, or behavioral classes, or they could be Mild Intellectual Disability classes, or Developmental Disability classes.

When the IPRC establishes exceptionalities for your child, they can set one exceptionality (i.e. behavioral, or learning disability), or they can set dual exceptionality (i.e. Learning Disability and Behavioral, or Behavioral and Emotional).

Taking This To Your School

Please remember that the structure of the committees described above may be different than the ones that are present in your particular school or school board. The point of this section is that you can take the *principles* of this section and apply them to your school. Talk to a teacher, a vice-principal, a special education teacher or someone at the school who is willing to help you to understand the particular approaches, committees and opportunities at your school for your child. Also, a parent support group can be very helpful. There will be parents there who have gone through it before, and they can help you to navigate through the school system to get the best help for your child.

A Note About Psychological Testing

Psychological testing (which can also be referred to as psychoeducational testing) is testing which must be done by a psychologist. The testing looks at the child's learning strengths and weaknesses. It generally looks at IQ (intellectual quotient), as well as academic achievement. IQ looks at your child's innate abilities for learning, thinking and problem solving. Academic achievement assesses what level your child is functioning at for the major school subjects—like reading, writing and mathematics.

Psychoeducational testing can establish your child's IQ, as well as establish if there is a learning disability present. If there is a learning disability, then it is important to get the help needed in the school system. Your child will qualify for support if he or she has a learning disability, irrespective of where you live. If your child has ADD and a Learning Disability, then your child will still qualify for support in areas which don't give support for ADD alone.

> **Ideally, every child or teen with ADD should have psychoeducational testing.**

This relates to the fact that approximately 40 percent of kids and teens with ADD also have learning differences or learning disabilities. In all other areas of medicine, when there is a co-existing condition that occurs that frequently, we always test for it. In this case, however, psychological testing is not always done— and this relates to the cost and insurance coverage.

Psychoeducational testing is quite costly. While it may vary where you live, it generally costs in the range of $1500 to $2000. Insurance may not pay for it. School systems are able to provide psychological testing, though they often have too few psychologists, and insufficient funding to test all of the kids that ideally would be tested. In the area that I work, there are many children who do not even get onto the list for psychological testing, and if they do, they often wait one to two years to get the testing. If you do decide to get testing done "privately" (i.e. you pay for it yourself), then you can take it back to the school, and they can use the results to go to an IPRC, create an IEP, and start the process of helping your child academically.

A Final Word About IEP's

It's important that you are aware that an IEP is a contract between you and the school. If the school has put something into writing for the IEP (i.e. they say that your child will get two hours of support per week) and they aren't delivering it, a quick discussion with the principal will fix that. If it doesn't, you can easily go "up the ladder" in the school's administration to ensure that the accommodations and modifications in the IEP are being met.

The school knows that the IEP is a written contract that must be honored, however, most parents don't realize the strength and importance of the IEP. This is why many schools will put general, non-specific supports in place for the IEP, rather than including specific details. They don't do this in an effort to NOT provide support to students, rather they have limited resources, and they want to make sure that they can meet the needs of all of the students with the resources that they have.

My advice to parents regarding IEPs is as follows:

1.   Get an ally in the school—i.e. a special education teacher, a teacher, etc. who can help you out.

2.   Get clear about which accommodations and/or modifications would be helpful to your son or daughter.

3.   Listen to the advice of the professionals who have assessed your child/teen about what can be helpful for him or her.

4.   Talk to parents from a parent support group about what has been helpful for their kids—particularly in your school board— (though be careful of parents who have become too negative, which can happen sometimes).

5.   Use this book and other resources to brainstorm other strategies which may be helpful to your son or daughter.

6. Be kind, cooperative and helpful with the school before setting up the IEP (i.e. don't pick fights with them over how they are handling your child). Take the position of being an understanding, concerned parent, who is concerned about your own child, and also the well being of all of the students of the school.

7. Attend the IPRC; provide input into the IEP.

8. Consider inviting the Psychologist, or Psychiatrist to attend the meeting to ensure that the best strategies are included to help your son or daughter. In some communities, you may also be able to find an "academic advocate," who has expertise in helping kids with ADD and/or learning disabilities get the help they need from the school board. N.B. If you can't find one, search for an ADD coach in your community. He or she may either be able to help you, or point you in the right direction.

9. Once the IEP is written, you can hold the school accountable to what they have agreed upon if they do not provide the resources that they have put into the IEP.

These nine steps are suggested, based on my experience working with many families over my years in practice. When things are going well with the school, then there is less concern, and these steps will just be helpful for you to be thorough. However, when there are problems and challenges—these steps can make a huge difference in achieving a good outcome for your son or daughter.

I have seen many families over the years where the situation with the school became negative, and, frankly, nasty. The parents felt that the school was not being understanding or helpful, and this was worsening things for their son or daughter. And while these parents were likely "right," the ultimate goal is to get the best help in place for their child, and they need to cooperate with the school.

In this case, being helpful, supportive and cooperative (see #6 above) can help to change the nature of the relationship with the school. This helps the school to give more support and help than they were previously. Then once the IEP is written, with many helpful suggestions in it, the parent now has something "in writing" which he/she can use to hold the school accountable to meet their child's needs.

Accommodations vs. Modifications

When discussing what the school can do to help you out, it is important for you to understand the difference between accommodations and modifications. Accommodations refer to the fact that your child is still expected to do the same quality and quantity of academic work, though they are going to get some accommodations to make it easier for them to accomplish it (i.e. taking tests in a quiet room, for example).

Modifications, on the other hand, involve actually changing the academic requirements expected of your child. When a curriculum is modified, your child is no longer meeting the regular academic requirements in the same way that the other students in their grade are meeting them. When you are reviewing options for an IEP, be clear about whether the school is recommending accommodations or modifications, and be clear about what the implications will be for your child's education over time.

Strategies To Help Your Child With His/Her Education

In this section, we are going to cover specific strategies which will be helpful to your son or daughter with ADD. Some of these will help whether they are formally worked into an IEP, or whether they are just done by yourself, with some help from the teacher.

Behavioral Control in September

At the start of a school year, it is important for September to be about establishing behavioral control. If teachers focus too much on academics before giving your ADD child a chance to get used to the new class and new routine, then that will make it harder for your child to succeed. Have a discussion with the teacher at the beginning of the school year about how important it is for your child to get a chance to "get used to" the new school year and new expectations.

Seating Arrangements

In the classroom, it is best if the students sit in a "traditional" seating arrangement. This means that all of the desks are facing toward the teacher. In this type of seating arrangement, all students are facing forward, and it is best for the ADD student to be sitting near the front of the class. This relates to the fact that it will be much easier for the student to stay focused on the school work when they are facing forward, and much easier to focus when he is not looking at four rows of other students before seeing the teacher.

Some teachers have a preference of putting kids into a "group" seating arrangement, where students are facing other students and they can only partially see the teacher. While this may be helpful for some pedagogical goals, it can be very distracting for the ADD student. Ask the teacher if it is possible to have a traditional seating arrangement, and if not, can the ADD student sit close to the teacher. Sitting close to the teacher can make a big difference on its own.

Workload

When it comes to the workload, your ADD child may need an adjustment. It is very important that ADD students receive help and support to break assignments into smaller, more manageable steps.

It is very common for ADD students to get overwhelmed, and then stop working. If they can learn early on, that they need to break work down into small steps, then they can become more productive. (The answer to old saying of "How do you eat an elephant?" seems appropriate here: "One bite at a time.")

Initially, students may need help from a teacher, parent or tutor to break down the assignment into smaller tasks, and help to make sure that each task is completed well. This also creates "mini deadlines," which can be helpful for time management of bigger projects.

Time management for people with ADD can often be a challenge. People with ADD often classify time as either: a) *now*, or b) *not now*. ADD students often struggle because when the book report is assigned for a due date three weeks from now, it is classified as "not now." However, the night before, it is "now" and a panic ensues. This is why it is so important to set mini deadlines for the work which was broken into smaller pieces. That way, reading the first five chapters and taking notes is completed in five days, and then the next five chapters and notes are due five days later, etc.

Some ADD students will need an adjustment in the amount of work assigned. In other words, she may do better when she is not required to do all of the repetition that is normally assigned to all of the other students.

Productivity and then Accuracy

It's important for the ADD student to get support in becoming productive. The efforts of the teacher and parent should initially be on the student becoming productive. If they aren't accurate in the beginning, don't focus too much on that. Make sure that he is actually producing work, and developing good work habits. Once these are in place, *then* focus more on accuracy. In the beginning, if he feels that he is being criticized too much, this can lower his motivation to produce the work, and then this can negatively impact his school work production.

Parent Teacher Communication

We covered earlier how important it is for parents and teachers to communicate well to support your son or daughter. How does that work on a day-to-day basis?

One of the best ways to do this is with a student notebook that goes back and forth with your son or daughter. This can be an "agenda"—where your son writes down the day's homework and notes for parents, or it can be a parent-teacher communication book—where the only ones writing in it are the parent and the teacher.

Many schools encourage the students to use an agenda. If this is the case in your school, you may need to set up a plan where the teacher (or an educational assistant) can help to make sure that your son has written in it all that he is supposed to. Because the agenda isn't helpful if the student doesn't write down what is supposed to go in the book.

In this day and age, some teachers and parents agree to do daily updates via email. This method of communication can work well, though you'll have to coordinate with the teacher to see if it can work in your specific situation (i.e. some teachers don't like to check email daily). If you do use email, just remember these points about emails:

1. Sometimes email messages don't get through.

2. Sometimes important email messages end up in the spam folder.

3. Emails are not confidential—so be cautious about the nature of the information which is being sent over email.

One other important aspect of help that the teacher can provide is making sure that your daughter comes home with the right books and materials in her backpack. Parent teacher communication doesn't work if your daughter forgot the communication book at school, and homework doesn't get done if the textbook is at school as well. This is a basic habit that will be important for your daughter to develop, though in the beginning, it is important that she receive help to make sure that this happens.

Homework

While schools vary in the amount of homework they send home, there generally is homework assigned, and the amount tends to increase as the years progress.

I generally recommend less homework in grades one through six. This is particularly important for an ADD child who has been struggling, and then issues come up at home with homework completion. If homework is a struggle, then talk to the teacher about adjusting the amount of work expected from your child. Be clear that I am not saying that your child should be exempt from homework, rather, an adjustment of the amount of homework could be helpful.

One issue which comes up over and over again is that ADD kids may not complete their classroom work, and the teacher sends that work home as extra homework. Then, the student has the 20 minutes of assigned homework, plus an extra 30 minutes because he didn't finish the schoolwork in class that day. I strongly recommend that parents talk to the teacher about making sure that the student completes his classroom work in class, and not sending that work home. If the student can't get the work done in class, then strategies need to be developed to help with work completion in class. Homework at night can be challenging enough for parents without extra classroom work being "piled on."

When it comes to homework completion at home, it is critically important to set up a routine. Most families make the mistake of deciding each day when to start homework. Think about it—do you have to think about brushing your teeth in the morning? For every adult that I've ever spoken to about this—they can clearly say that no matter how tired they are, or how little sleep they got—they brush their teeth in the morning after getting up.

Why does it work on "auto-pilot"? Because it's a routine—a habit. Once you did that for days and weeks, you got so used to it, that you didn't have to think about it anymore. Let's harness the power of a routine into a homework routine, so that there won't be challenges and battles each evening, rather, you'll have a habit that is easy to continue.

I generally recommend that parents set up a homework routine with their child's input. The homework routine can be something like this:

- Get home at 3:30 pm.

- Have a snack.

- Watch one TV show (or go play outside for 30 minutes).

- Meet with mom at the kitchen table at 4 pm.

- Open the agenda/parent teacher communication book, and review the work that has to be done.

- Plan for the time that will be needed for each task.

- Get out a timer, and say: "Now you're going to do your math questions for the next 11 minutes. Work hard on them until the clock beeps. Do you think you can get all of the questions on page 32 done in that time?"

- Finish the homework with praise and accolades for the job well done.

The parent needs to supervise the homework. Sometimes this means sitting with your son and helping with specific learning tasks. Sometimes it just means helping to make sure that your son doesn't get distracted, and stays on task. Be careful to remain positive during homework, and don't get frustrated and upset. This is one of the reasons that using a timer can be so helpful.

Using a timer is a great strategy for ADD kids. It can be a kitchen timer, or a digital timer. This part doesn't matter (And of course, you don't have to buy your child the newest iPod touch so that he can have a timer to use for homework).

Why do timers work? They work for several reasons. People with ADD often have trouble with time management. When you use a timer, you are "externalizing" time. This means that you are taking the time out of the person's mind, and making it outside of them—i.e. external. This in and of itself can be helpful. Timers also create mini-deadlines. Deadlines can be very helpful, because they help students finish a task on time (i.e. it becomes "now" rather than "not-now"). Timers can also stimulate a fun/challenging component - i.e. a "beat the clock" game. Beat the clock can be that you gradually increase the amount of time that the timer is set for (i.e. "You did nine minutes yesterday; do you think you can do 10 minutes today?). Or it can be used to see how much work is done in the time available (i.e. "You did 10 problems yesterday in nine minutes, do you think you can do 11 today?"). Of course, when playing "beat the clock," be careful not to sacrifice accuracy for speed. This can be an issue for some kids, so be mindful of this.

Restlessness In The Classroom

It's great if the teacher can set up the ability for your child to move a little during the course of the regular school day. Often times, ADD kids feel contained, or trapped during the school day. If the teacher lets her help handing out papers, or asks her to take something down to the office, then that can let your daughter clear off some of her extra energy so that she can be productive in the class academically.

Because movement can be so helpful for ADD kids, it is important that they do not lose recess or sports as a punishment. This is not to say that they are to be allowed to go out for recess or to sports with no exceptions—though I encourage parents and teachers to find other solutions for consequences if at all possible.

This relates to the fact that when ADD students are taken out of the physical exercise that they need, it can make the problems in the classroom even worse, because the student is feeling trapped, and he hasn't had an outlet for his energy.

There are some "fidget toys" which may be helpful to your child or teen. In my office, I have a few boxes of toys for kids to play with. One of the favorite genres of toys are the *transformers*. These are great toys for playing, and to use one's hands. There are many parents who will tell their kids or teens to stop playing with the toys while they are talking to me. And I always correct the parents—explaining that their son or daughter is able to pay attention better when they have something to fidget with, rather than if they put that object down. This rule doesn't apply 100 percent of the time, but it is generally the case. There are several products which are considered "fidget toys" which can be used in the classroom without disturbing other children. Talk to the teacher about these before making a financial investment in them.

Music While Learning

Many ADD students, particularly teenagers, can learn better if they have the ability to listen to their music while they work. While many parents and educators want to stop the child or teen from listening to their music, it is often easier for an ADD student to do one thing, if he can pay attention to more than one thing, i.e. he can focus on homework better if he can listen to music as well. This doesn't apply 100 percent of the time, so it is fair for you to tell your son that you are going to do a trial, to see if he is more productive with homework if he is wearing his headset. If he is less productive, then you take away the ability to use the headset.

I have had times in my office when I write a note to the school requesting that a patient of mine be given the right to listen to headphones during quiet work times to help the student's productivity.

Teaching Styles That Work

ADD students do much better with animated and interactive teachers. They do better with teaching styles which are much more active and participatory. While it is not generally possible to have teachers change their teaching style in the middle of the school year, it is important to consider this when working with the school to find the right teacher for your daughter for next year. Also, you may be able to have input into which educational assistant your son works with, or which tutor he has.

It is best if the teachers do the most challenging work in the morning. Everybody has a better attention span in the morning and it gradually worsens through the course of the day. This is even more pronounced in kids with ADD. To the extent that the teacher is able to do this, it will help your child or teen.

It is also helpful if the teacher intersperses high appeal activities with low appeal activities—i.e. we will get to do drama after we finish math. This can help your son's motivation to get through the harder work.

Transition Planning

Kids and teens with ADD often struggle with transitions. They may have trouble with disengaging from one activity and moving toward another. It is very important for teachers, tutors and parents to be aware of this and to plan accordingly.

ADD students often need regular reminders that the activity will be changing shortly. Reminders like: "Ten more minutes until we stop and move on—seven more minutes—four more minutes—two more minutes—Okay, now it's time to stop and move on to the next thing."

Not only will this help the student to realize that he needs to wrap up and move on; more importantly, it can also prevent a major meltdown from happening. Some ADD students get very angry and upset if they feel that there were forced to stop doing something before they were finished.

These principles of planning for transitions apply in the classroom as well as at home.

Clear Classroom Expectations

It is very helpful if the teacher can have very clear expectations of classroom behavior and requirements. Having these rules/expectations posted in the class is ideal. It is far better that the rules be clear to all students, and not let the ADD student feel that he is being singled out, and treated differently. If the teacher can articulate all of the expectations to all of the students, then this can be avoided, and it can help the ADD student to comply with the classroom routines.

Token or Reward Systems

It can be very helpful for an ADD student if a teacher is able to establish, or already uses a token system. If the student earns credits, stickers, or "funny money," then he can be quite motivated to complete the tasks requested of him. When this type of system is done well, it can be very positive for all of the students.

Activities which can be rewarded include: getting your agenda signed by your parent each day, homework completion, helping out other students (encouraging pro-social behavior), working quietly during desk time, etc.

Often teachers will set up a time to allow students to "redeem" their credits. This could be as simple as getting a toy from the dollar store for 10 credits. It can also be elaborate—like an auction at the end of the term—where the teachers get parents to donate old books and toys, and then the kids can bid using their credits to buy the toys.

Daily Behavior Report Card

Younger students may do well with active monitoring of their daily behavior and functioning. This can be set up as its own reward system.

Generally, a daily behavior report card will need its own binder or notebook. It includes the teacher rating the student multiple times per day about his functioning in several realms. For younger students, the scoring may be a happy face for a good result, a neutral face for a fine result, and a frowning face for a poor result. For an older student, a score of one to seven can be used, where one is needs improvement, and seven is outstanding.

Here is a sample daily behavior report card. In this sample, the student is measured in seven different subjects or time points in the day. The teacher (or teachers) add their scoring in each section, and then initial the bottom.

SUBJECTS	1	2	3	4	5	6	7
Follows Rules							
Gets Class Work Done							
Gets Along Well With Others							
Teacher's Initials							

Table 3: Sample daily behavior report card

Feel free to create your own version of this daily behavior report card, based on the principles of this one. You can change what is measured based on what is best for your son's situation, and you can change the number of measurement points.

It is clear that this kind of approach requires significant work and cooperation with the teacher. Be sure to talk with the teacher during the planning stages of this approach, to make sure that it turns into a helpful approach, and increases communication between yourself as the parent, and the teacher.

This strategy would not generally work well with a teenager, though some teens do have to get a sheet signed by each teacher. This can relate to a student who has had chronic absences or "lates." In this case, it may be required that the high-school student have each teacher sign an attendance sheet to prove that the student attended each class or was on time. The student may be on "contract," i.e. agreeing to comply with the attendance or punctuality rules in order to continue on at school.

The Punishment Hierarchy

Many students will get into a situation where they have earned some sort of punishment at school. It is important with an ADD student that the teacher not get into multiple punishments, and in a way which is very negative, leading to problems and lost productivity.

It is best if punishment starts out as mild, direct and private. This is opposed to harsh and public. Any student does poorly when he feels that he is being singled out in front of all of his peers.

It is also important for consequences to be handled quickly—i.e. "swift justice." This relates to the fact that if the teacher waits until later to address an issue, this often takes away the real learning for the student.

A "task table" can be helpful. This is a desk where the student can go and do one or many sheets of extra school work for the misbehavior.

When it comes to suspensions, I generally recommend that the school do in-school suspensions. This takes away the sense of a "holiday" from school because of misbehavior. If your child does get a suspension from school, it is important that he or she does not get a "holiday day" at home, sitting and watching TV and playing Xbox. It is important that you ensure that your child has to do reading, school work, or just sit quietly until school hours are over.

Tips for Teens at School

Teens with ADD can have their own challenges with high school. In high school, the expectations are much higher and the structure around the student is much lower. This can create a challenge for the ADD teen.

Teens need to develop habits that serve them well. Using a daytimer, agenda, or even a technological solution to keep track of their daily assignments and upcoming deadlines is critical.

Teens with ADD can be helped significantly by an academic mentor. This is a teacher, educational assistant, or even a school administrator who just checks in with the student daily or weekly, to check on how things are going, and to monitor workload, deadlines, and other school challenges which may come up. This can help with school productivity, help to teach organizational and learning skills and it can also prevent crises from happening.

Some schools have a learning strategies course that students can take as a one credit course. This teaches strategies for successful academic performance, and can make a big difference for a student's functioning. Ask your school if it is available for your son or daughter.

Using technology can make a big difference for teens with ADD. Using a laptop or netbook to take notes can help a lot. Your son will need to learn keyboarding, and will need to get permission from the school to do this.

Recording school classes can be helpful as well. There are many digital recorders available now that can record classes, and then the recordings can be downloaded onto the computer or MP3 player. This can help students who learn best by listening and repetition. You will need the teacher's permission to record the classes.

Consider Bucks for B's: This is a simple concept—consider rewarding your teen with money for getting decent grades, or for showing improvement. As a doctor, I have heard many parents' objections to this concept—mostly: "Isn't this bribery?" Often times, these same parents give their kids five dollars per goal scored on the hockey rink. Is it bribery? I guess so—but it's not negative if it is helping your daughter achieve a goal which is helpful to her and helpful to her education.

Study Buddy: It is very helpful if a teen can partner up with a study buddy. This student can meet with your son regularly, to help each other to stay on task and to get work done.

Get Contact Information for other students: It can be helpful for your teen to get contact info from other students to get work that is missed, or homework assignments from days missed. Even though teachers should help in this area, sometimes it is overlooked, and having another student's contact info can help a lot.

Sometimes teachers will hold after-school, help sessions. These can be extremely helpful, and I encourage ADD students to take advantage of them as much as possible.

Good Communication: Finally, it is worthwhile for parents to have good communication with the high school teachers, hopefully including regular parent teacher meetings. These could be every six weeks, so that the parents are aware of the progress being made and any issues arising. It is important that your teen be invited to these meetings, and it is also important that these meetings occur even if your teen doesn't attend, or doesn't want the meetings to happen.

A Quiet Room for Tests

This applies whether we are talking about kids or teens—having a quiet environment for tests can make a big difference. If a student is in a large classroom, the little noises of pages turning, or someone tapping a pencil can be very distracting for an ADD student, and can lead to poor performance on a test. Schools generally have another, quieter environment where the student can write the test.

Extra Time for Tests

Some ADD individuals may do better with extra time for tests. This will allow them to get the information they have in their heads out onto the paper, without undue pressure taking away their ability to perform. This accommodation may require more approval than the teacher is able to provide, and should be discussed with the special education teacher, or the school administration.

Nurture Your Child or Teen's Interests or Passions

Many students with ADD have one or two subjects that are much harder for them, and one or two subjects which come more easily. In high school, kids with ADD can feel that subjects just have no relevance to them, and they aren't interested (the classic question: How is this history class relevant to my life?). In the early years of education, there are so many mandatory requirements that it can be hard for an ADD student who struggles in a particular area. However, when he or she gets to high school, in particular the later years of high school, it can be easier for him to choose subjects he likes. And we know that anyone with ADD focuses much better on subjects that he likes.

While many educators spend a lot of time helping students with their weaknesses—which is necessary—I encourage you as a parent to help to nurture your son or daughter's strengths. If they are great at photography, see if you can get enriching classes or activities outside of school. If they love writing, or geography, or something else, encourage them, and celebrate any success that they have dramatically. Your enthusiastic support can make a big difference. You can also reassure your child that when he gets far enough in school, he won't have to take math anymore, and he can take a lot more of the arts (or whatever his area of interest is). And if he goes to a post-secondary school, he can focus exactly on what it is he loves (i.e. college for photography, graphic design, writing, etc.).

Beware of the Negative Halo

It is all too common in my office to see kids and teens who have been given a "negative halo" at school. This refers to the fact that they have gotten into trouble so many times that the school now expects them to get into trouble all of the time. If anything goes wrong, they consider your son or daughter to be a part of it. It's like your child is wearing a halo, but instead of it glowing like an angel, it is dark, like a..., let's just say, "trouble maker."

If you are reading this book before your child has gotten into trouble with the school, the strategies listed above will help to ensure that you can avoid this negative halo from developing.

If your son or daughter already has this negative halo in place, then you have a lot of work to do to help to undo this. And it is critically important that you do. It can be very hard for an ADD child or teen to succeed when they feel that everyone sees them in a negative light.

How do you turn around a negative halo?

Firstly, you need to reframe the difficulties that your child has been experiencing. By introducing the diagnosis of ADD and/or learning disabilities, this can help. This helps the school to understand that your child is not just being "bad," rather there is a medical condition which needs help.

If your child is already diagnosed (and the school knows about it), you need to get more help from professionals—either your doctor, psychologist, or even a tutor. Specifically, you need to develop a new understanding of what is going on for your child, and which strategies can make a difference to help. This book can even be the resource to give you new understandings and new strategies to move forward with the school.

Explain to the school that you are very concerned with how things are going, because they just don't seem to be working for your child.

Explain to the school, that based on your discussions with your doctor, or based on insights you've received from reading, or from a parent support group, you believe that there are challenges that your child is experiencing that are not being addressed. Then discuss the approaches which you believe will make a difference.

Remember that members of the school staff are educators and experts in their fields. Ask them for the solutions that they recommend. See if they can bring in other professionals to help out—i.e. the school psychologist or social worker who may help bring a fresh perspective and help to improve things.

Once you have reframed the problems and are moving forward together with a new approach, realize that it will take time to remove the negative halo. If your son has one good week, the school will still be concerned about things going wrong. If he has three good weeks, they start to believe that this may be a turnaround. Once a certain amount of time has passed (and this amount can vary a lot based on the school and the individuals involved), the school will stop considering your child to have a negative halo. Just realize that it takes a while for a negative halo to develop, and it probably takes longer for a negative halo to be "removed."

A Comment about Private Schools

Some parents try to enroll their child with ADD into a private school, hoping that it will make a big difference. All I can say from experience is that the response is often variable. Some private schools do not have the resources to help kids with ADD to get the help they need. Other families have been told that they cannot enroll their child with ADD in the school this year, as the school has too many kids with ADD already, and they won't be able to help.

There are some private schools which are created specifically to help kids and teens with ADD (and/or learning disabilities). They are designed to help, and they can make a big difference. Of course, private schools can be extremely costly, particularly if they are developed to meet a specific need—i.e. ADD or learning disabilities.

In summary, we have covered a lot of different aspects of ADD in school. This chapter has covered the challenges which may come up in school, the processes built into the school to handle issues, as well as specific strategies that can be used to increase your child's chances for success. The best way to start with this section, is to choose one or two strategies that you think will be helpful, and work on them. Once you find out if those strategies are successful, go ahead and try other strategies. Go through this step by step and persist—your child is counting on you for your help.

If after you try the school strategies discussed here, you aren't getting the results you need, I encourage you to read a book by Dr. Peter Jensen, called: *Making The System Work For Your Child With ADHD*. In this book, Dr. Jensen combines his extensive knowledge and research background with input from parents who were "in the trenches" to give you great approaches to get the help that you need for your child at school (as well as in other areas too).

CHAPTER 7

Step 5: Medication Treatment for ADD

■

I f your son or daughter has been diagnosed with ADD, then the discussion about medication will certainly happen. That discussion may start with the doctor, but it will be a long term conversation—often including many other people—people like your neighbor, your mother-in-law, or your well meaning Aunt Sally. You may review scientific information and advice from your doctor, to make a decision to try a medication. And then a new news report about side effects or problems could rock your confidence about using a medication and you may want to stop. This chapter will review the science behind medications for ADD, and help you to understand the major issues about using medications for ADD.

Why does every doctor who diagnoses ADD end up having a discussion about medication with his/her patient? Because, to date, there is very strong scientific data demonstrating that medications work. There have been literally thousands of children and teens who have participated in well-designed clinical trials which show that ADD medications are helpful and safe.

Why do medications for ADD remain so controversial?

Medications for ADD seem controversial, because it is always a difficult decision to decide to start your child or teen on a medication for a psychiatric

111

or mental health issue. Our society has significant stigma around psychiatric and mental health issues, so people don't understand, and they judge very quickly. People also have the illusion that they understand the nature of ADD, because they get distracted too, sometimes—but when they try harder they do fine. They have no concept of what ADD is truly like.

And then there are always news stories about the dangers or problems with medication. It's my belief that if there is a "slow news day," and the newspapers or TV shows are eager to increase their readership or viewership, they run a story like: "Don't Drug Your Children," and they achieve their goals. This of course makes it much harder for parents of kids and teens to stick with their educated decision to use medications for ADD.

How Do We Know that ADD Medications Work?

As mentioned above, there have been numerous studies which have had literally thousands of kids and teens enrolled as subjects. These studies are set up as *randomized, double blind, placebo controlled trials*. This means that once the child is entered into the study (with a diagnosis of ADD), then he is *randomized* to receive either the active medication for ADD, or a *placebo*. The placebo is an inactive substance which will have no impact on the ADD symptoms.

The placebo is also put into a pill or capsule that looks identical to the active medicine, so that it is impossible for the patient, parent, doctor or even the pharmacist to know whether the patient is receiving active medicine or placebo. This is what is meant by the fact that the study is *double blind*. That means that the patients don't know what they are getting, and neither does the doctor/researcher. This setup helps to eliminate bias. If the parents, patients and doctors don't know if they are getting active medicine or placebo, then their own beliefs about which one should work can't impact on the outcome of the study.

Generally ADD studies are set up for four to eight weeks. The researchers complete questionnaires and actively monitor the subject's response to the treatment they are taking.

After the study is completed, the researchers "break the code" and find out which patients took active medicine and which took the placebo/control medicine. They then analyze the response to treatment, comparing the active medicine group to the placebo group. It is very common for the ADD medication group to have had a great response to treatment, whereas the placebo group has minimal response. The statisticians of the study review the data and decide if the results are found to be due to chance, or due to a difference between the active treatment and placebo. In just about every study for ADD medications, there is a strong medication response, which is deemed to be far better than the response to placebo.

As a clinician who works with ADD regularly, and having read many studies about medications for ADD, it is fair to say that the response rates for medication in this condition are around 60 to 80 percent. This is a very robust response, and means that most people who take medication for ADD will benefit.

How Does Medication Treatment Fit With All of the Other Treatments?

Probably the best study done for the treatment of ADD is called the Multimodal Treatment Study[1]. It is often referred to as the MTA. In the MTA, the researchers took 579 children with ADD, and put them through 14 months of treatment. This was done at multiple research sites. The study was completed in the late 1990s. It was designed to look at whether medication treatment, behavioral treatment or both would be best for ADD.

---

1   A 14-month randomized clinical trial of treatment strategies for attention-deficit/ hyperactivity disorder. The MTA Cooperative Group, "Multimodal Treatment Study of Children with ADHD", *Arch Gen Psychiatry. 1999 Dec; 56 (12): 1073-86.*

The MTA study compared the response of kids with ADD to one of four treatment groups:

1. Medication treatment only: this group received Ritalin® (methylphenidate) medication three times per day—i.e. morning, noon and late afternoon. Their medicine dose was set accurately at the beginning of the study, and then they were monitored for 14 months. Please note that this was short-acting medicine; the new generation of long acting medicines hadn't been developed yet.

2. Intensive Behavioral treatment: This treatment included intensive treatment with parent, child and school components. There was significant intensity, and the number of hours was far beyond what one can generally get in most communities to help with ADD.

3. A combination of Medication treatment and Intensive Behavioral Treatment.

4. Community care: this group of kids received the regular treatment that their own doctor in their own community provided. They would come to the research center for regular monitoring, though they wouldn't receive any active treatment from the study.

At the end of the 14 months, the researchers looked at the rate of response of the children to the different treatments. Surprisingly, the "community treatment" group only had about 25 percent of children who were deemed to be a clinical success. In this group, approximately two thirds had taken medication. The "intensive behavioral treatment" group had a 34 percent response to treatment—those patients were deemed clinical successes.

The "medication only" group had a 56 percent response to treatment, and the combination group of "medication plus behavioral treatment" had a 68 percent response.

When the researchers analyzed the statistics of the results, they found that although there was some difference between the medication-only group, and the combination treatment group, this was not statistically significant. The significant difference was between the groups which had the study protocol for medicine in their treatment (i.e. medication only and combination treatment), and the groups which didn't (community care and behavioral treatment only).

This study shows that when medication is used in the treatment of ADD, and it is done to a higher standard of monitoring, it can produce very strong results, which are better than behavioral treatment on its own.

Although statistically, there was no significant difference between the medication only and the combination treatment group, there were several measures in which the combination group did better. These included: oppositional or aggressive behavior, teacher-rated social skills, parent-child relations, reading achievement, and internalizing symptoms (this refers to feelings of sadness or anxiety).

This study has clearly shown that *having combination treatment for ADD is the best approach*. Having a combination of medication and therapy yields the best results.

As a doctor working with patients in my office, I can clearly see that when people take medication without getting any therapy, they are missing a major component to the treatment. The saying that "pills don't teach skills" comes to mind. In other words, if the medication helps to control the inattention and hyperactivity/impulsivity, but the child doesn't have any coping skills to handle difficult situations, then he does not do as well as he can. And the flip side applies as well—if I see people who are going for therapy, and not trying medication—there can be struggles where the child has trouble implementing and following through on the skills being taught because of the untreated inattention, hyperactivity and impulsivity. When medication and therapy are used together, better outcomes can come from it.

Are ADD Medications Over-prescribed?

One of the topics which comes out in the press regularly is the fact that ADD medications are over-prescribed. You have to be careful about your son or daughter being put on these medications when they don't need them. These articles usually reference the fact that the pharmaceutical companies are trying to control the medical system or some variation of this claim.

When I look at what is going on for ADD treatment, there is an interesting paradox that I see. The ADD medications are both over- prescribed, and under-prescribed! You may wonder how this is possible.

In some communities, there are doctors who diagnose ADD very quickly, and write prescriptions before doing a thorough assessment. In these communities, the medications are over-prescribed. In other communities, there are too many barriers to getting good treatment, and ADD is under-diagnosed, and under-treated. In this case, the ADD medications are under-prescribed.

How do you protect against this? If you will, follow the advice in Step 2 about ensuring that a proper diagnosis is made, you will have the confidence that your child is properly diagnosed. When this is the case, you have protected against getting a prescription unnecessarily.

And if you have any questions, be sure to ask your doctor. Make sure that you are satisfied with the answers before you proceed. If you need to, get a second opinion.

The Main Way To Decide About ADD Medications

When you are faced with making a decision about whether to use ADD medications or not, you may not know how to make the decision. In other words, you may not have criteria to help you to make a decision, or the certainty to know if you are making the right decision. Many people "sleep on it" to see if their "gut" can tell them if it is the right decision. Or they just feel overwhelmed and feel guilty about trying medicine... or feel guilty about *not* trying medicine!

Based on my reading of the research and working with many families, it is my advice that the best way to decide when it is time to use a medication is this: balancing the risk-benefit ratio.

When you need to make the decision about using an ADD medication, you need to balance the risks versus the benefits.

As was mentioned above, approximately 60 to 80 percent of people have a good response to medication for ADD. This is a very high percentage, and shows strong benefits.

Generally speaking, approximately 10 to 15 percent of people develop side effects to medications which are a problem. Some people may get "nuisance side effects," which can be managed, but some people get side effects which are not manageable.

So, on face value, the risk benefit ratio in ADD is that there is a 60 to 80 percent chance of benefit, and a 10 to 15 percent chance of risks. This suggests that it would be a good idea to try an ADD medication.

Your job, when you are considering a medicine for your son or daughter, is to talk about the specifics of your child's treatment. Maybe there are certain factors which may change the risk benefit ratio in his or her case. For example, if you have a son who did great on Concerta˚, and your daughter is now diagnosed with ADD, your doctor may believe that your daughter has more than an 80 percent chance of responding to this same medicine. Or perhaps your son has a tic disorder, and your doctor believes that the risks are higher than 10 to 15 percent, because the tics could be worsened by certain medicines.

While considering taking a medication for ADD, it is important to remember the "flip side" of the risk benefit ratio. This relates to the fact that there are risks if you don't treat ADD effectively. Kids and teens with untreated ADD are at higher risk of:

- Academic underachievement,
- Drug and alcohol problems,
- Low self esteem, depression and anxiety,

- Social problems,

- Family problems, and

- Driving accidents (when old enough to drive).

If you can treat ADD safely and effectively, then you can significantly lower these risks, and improve longer term outcomes for your son or daughter.

Using Impairment As a Deciding Factor

Remember that we referred to the fact that impairment is critical to the diagnosis of ADD in Step 2. In other words, if there is no impairment in your child's life, then there is no real disorder. It is important to remember this when considering a medication. When there is impairment from ADD which is interfering with your son or daughter's functioning in any realm (like academic, social, emotional or psychological), then it is worth considering medication to help to fix the impairment and help to get your child's life back on track.

Please realize that ongoing impairment will have an impact that can be long lasting. And that treating ADD earlier can make a difference in longer term outcomes.

Using Severity As A Deciding Factor

When a doctor assesses any patient for ADD, the doctor has a good sense as to whether the ADD is mild, moderate or severe in that particular individual. And the severity of the disorder can have a big impact on making decisions for treatment.

For example, if a child has mild ADD, and the parents are reluctant about using medication, and want to try therapy first, the doctor will likely agree (after providing education about the treatment options). The doctor will explain that he will want to monitor the response of the child to the non-medication treatments (i.e. "come back in three months and let's repeat the checklists"). And if the ADD gets worse, or the consequences of ADD become more concerning, then the doctor may push to use medications sooner.

If a child has severe ADD, which is causing significant impairment, then the doctor will likely suggest starting medicine much more quickly than if the disorder is mild and not causing so many concerns. To paraphrase what is written above, if the impairment is severe, then it is worth considering medication more quickly.

This discussion is similar to the discussion that many adults have with their doctor about blood pressure and medication. If there is borderline, or very mild high blood pressure, the doctor may say that it's time to start a blood pressure medicine. However, most adults are reluctant to start a medicine, so they beg their doctor, saying something like: "I just joined the gym. I'll go, and exercise, and lose weight like I'm supposed to. I'll take yoga, and meditate and de-stress."

And what does the doctor say to this? Usually something like: "Okay— but you need to come back in six weeks; then we need to see if you are making any progress... Because, if you aren't, we'll need to put you on the medicine because there are serious risks to not treating high blood pressure."

The same message applies to ADD. If the symptoms are mild, the doctor may agree with you to just monitor and add medicine later if needed. If the symptoms are more severe, then you may need to make the decision as soon as possible.

Remember, ADD Treatment is a Marathon, Not a Sprint

As you know, ADD lasts for months and years, not days or weeks. When you are working on treatment, you need to be prepared to work on ADD for the "long haul." When you think of treatment for ADD from the perspective of it being a marathon, not a sprint, you realize that you have to be comfortable with the decisions you make for the long term.

Be aware of this, particularly if you are working on the decision for medication. If you don't feel comfortable with your decision to start medication, and if you feel pressured by your doctor (or the teachers, etc.), then take more time to get the answers you need.

In my experience in my clinical practice, I see that when a parent is pushed too far too fast, they don't follow through with treatment in the long term. They may start medication and then stop after four weeks, and then not see the doctor for three years, because of the feelings of discomfort, or the feelings of being pushed.

It is important to get the answers you need, make informed decisions, and consider ADD treatment as a marathon, not a sprint. If you need more time to get answers, then say so—and take a reasonable amount of time. If the symptoms of your son or daughter are severe, then you may have less time to make your decision before more consequences come into effect, but make sure that you get the answers you need.

Realize that you have to pace yourself so that you can go the distance.

How Do ADD Medications Work?

ADD medications help boost the brain chemicals which are needed to improve inattention, hyperactivity and impulsivity. We have already discussed that people with ADD have brain differences compared to non-ADD controls (in research studies). It is often found that the frontal lobe—the part of the brain just behind the forehead—is mildly underactive in individuals with ADD. The frontal lobe is the area that is predominantly responsible for the executive functions—the higher level thinking and planning thoughts which help people to negotiate complex tasks.

To review how ADD medications work, we need to start with how one brain cell (neuron) communicates with another. The neurons have a long arm which carries an electrical signal toward the next cell. This is called an axon. When the signal gets to the end of the cell, there is a gap before the next cell, and this is called the synapse. For the message to move from one cell to the next, the electrical signal needs to be converted to a chemical signal, so that it may travel across the gap. The cell releases small chemical messengers to jump across the gap—and these are called neurotransmitters. When these neurotransmitters get to the other side, they bind to receptors on the receiving side of the next neuron, and that triggers the next cell to transmit the message.

After the neurotransmitter is released from the receptor, it is then "sucked up" by a recycle pump (called a transporter) on the first cell, so that it can be reused when another signal comes.

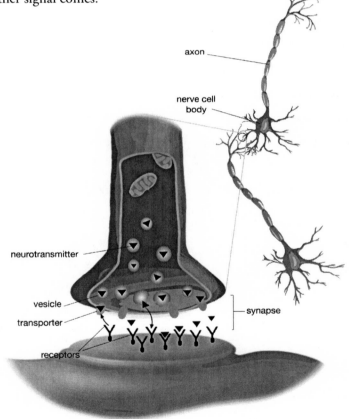

Image © Medical Integrity Inc.

FIGURE 1: One brain cell (neuron) communicating with another one

Now that we have established how the neurons communicate with one another, let's look at how the medications work.

When an ADD medication is taken, it crosses from the blood into the brain, and it goes to work right in the synapse. There it blocks the transporter which is intended to suck the neurotransmitter up after it has carried the signal to the next neuron. This means that there is more time that the neurotransmitter stays in the synapse; it has the effect of "turning up the volume" of the next signal (because the next signal triggers the presence of its own neurotransmitter in the synapse, as well as the neurotransmitter from the previous signal). When the amount of neurotransmitter is increased like that, it decreases ADD symptoms. When it comes to neurotransmitters in ADD, there are two which have been found to make the biggest difference in the treatment of ADD. They include: dopamine and norepinephrine (also referred to as noradrenaline in some countries).

While the medications have slightly different effects on each of these neurotransmitters, it is fair to say that when either or both dopamine and norepinephrine are increased, the symptoms of ADD decrease, thus improving functioning. Research has found that the different neurotransmitters have different effects on concentration. When dopamine is increased, it has the effect of increasing the volume of the signal that is being focused on. For example, the math homework page seems "louder," so it is easier to focus on. When norepinephrine is increased, it helps to dampen the noise. This means that if one is paying attention to math homework, one would be bothered less by the little noises around them. Obviously, if we could increase *both* dopamine and norepinephrine, there is a better chance that we can decrease ADD symptoms and improve functioning.

A good analogy to think about ADD neurotransmitters is an "old fashioned" radio. I don't mean the newer digital kind (where you turn the dial and the numbers move up one tenth increments on a digital dial). I am referring to the old kind, the one that had a red bar that you would move up and down the radio frequencies as you turned the dial. If you were trying to find a radio station on an old fashioned radio, you would have to scan through the frequencies, and find a signal that was coming through. You'd have to narrow in on the frequency to listen to that station.

You'd agree that to get good reception of that station, you'd need two components: a) a good, strong signal, and b) not too much static or noise at that spot on the dial.

The same applies to focusing in ADD. We need a "strong signal" to focus on, and we need "less noise" to be able to focus. In the example of the radio, the dopamine would increase the strength of the signal from the station, and the norepinephrine would lower the amount of static or noise on the dial.

When it comes to the array of ADD medications, they all work on the neurotransmitters, though slightly differently. When it comes to the stimulants in that array, the methylphenidate medicines, they have a strong effect on boosting dopamine, and a weaker effect on norepinephrine. The therapeutic amphetamines have a strong effect on both dopamine and norepinephrine, while the non-stimulant, Strattera, has a strong effect on norepinephrine, and a weaker effect on dopamine.

Even though this discussion may suggest that the therapeutic amphetamines may be the best medications for ADD (because they work strongly on both dopamine and norepinephrine), the reality is that the effect for any one individual is likely more dependent on their genetic makeup—i.e. the way their transporters are formed in the synapse, rather than solely on this explanation of how medicines work. Therefore, be sure to work with your doctor to find the best medicine for your son or daughter.

What Are the Medications For ADD?

When it comes time to consider a medication for ADD, it is important to know what is available. Your doctor will often discuss his or her best recommendation for you. Many—but not all— doctors will put that in the context of all of the treatments available. It's important for you to understand all of the options you have.

From an overview level, there are two main groups of ADD medications. They are:

1. The Stimulant medicines.
2. The Non-Stimulant medicines.

When considering medicines for ADD, it is important to realize that there are "first line" medicines, and there are second and third line medicines. The first line medicines are medicines which are approved for treatment of ADD. This means that the regulators (i.e. the FDA in the USA, and its equivalent in other countries) have approved the medicine for the treatment of ADD.

There are also the so-called second and third line medicines; these can be used if the first line medicines don't work. These are medicines which are not officially approved for ADD, but they can still be helpful. An example here is the antidepressant medicine, buproprion, (marketed as Wellbutrin XL). There is some evidence that it helps with ADD, though it is not officially approved for it.

Within the two medicine groups, there are really just two types of medicine in each:

- In the stimulant medicines, there are the methylphenidate medicines, and the therapeutic amphetamines.
- In the non-stimulant medicines, there are atomoxetine, and extended release guanfacine.

This is shown in Table 2 below:

STIMULANT MEDICATION	1. Methylphenidate
	2. Therapeutic Amphetamines
NON-STIMULANT MEDICATION	3. Atomoxetine
	4. Guanfacine Extended Release

Table 4: The first line medications for ADD

As Table 4 shows, there are only four medications which are approved for ADD in the United States of America. Most other countries have at least two, if not three of these medicines approved.

When you look at Table 4, you may wonder why there are so few first line medicines listed, when you know that there are so many different medicines available for the treatment of ADD.

The answer is, that of all of the medications which are available to treat ADD, they all can be considered to be in one of these four categories.

First Line Medicines		Examples	Duration of Action (approx.)
Stimulants:	1) Methylphenidate	Ritalin	4 hrs
		Methylphenidate	4 hrs
		Methylin	4 hrs
		Focalin	4 hrs
		Rubifen	4 hrs
		Ritalin SR	6 hrs
		Ritalin LA	8 hrs
		Biphentin	8 hrs
		Metadate CD	8 hrs
		Concerta	12 hrs
		Focalin XR	12 hrs
		Daytrana Patch	12 hrs
	2) Therapeutic Amphetamines	Dexedrine	4 hrs
		Dextroamphetamine	4 hrs
		Adderall	4 hrs
		Dexedrine Spansules	8 hrs
		Adderall XR	12 hrs
		Mixed Amphetamine salts XR	12 hrs
		Vyvanse	13 hrs
Non-Stimulants:	3) Atomoxetine	Strattera	up to 24 hrs
	4) Guanfacine	Intuniv	up to 24 hrs

TABLE 5: The different forms of first line medications for ADD

Table 5 lists many of the forms of medicine available for ADD, and you can see how they actually can be grouped into the four categories listed in Table 4.

When your doctor discusses medicine with you, he may recommend a particular medication as the best first option for you. Your doctor's decision may relate to his previous experience with that medication, or some aspect of your story which suggests you may do well with one medicine over the other. Since there are no blood tests or prior way to decide which medicine will work, you need to allow for some trial and error. In other words, when you choose a medicine with your doctor, start at a low dose, and then monitor carefully for the response, and for any side effects. The dosage then gets adjusted until you have a good response. If there are problems with the first medicine, then you may get switched to a second medicine. This is the trial and error process.

Here is where understanding what is shown in Table 4 and Table 5 can help you: If your doctor starts you on a methylphenidate medicine—let's say: Concerta˙. This is a version of the medication methylphenidate which can last up to 12 hours. If it works well for your daughter, then you carry on. If it works well, but she's up each night until 1:30 am, then you will likely want to stay in the same category of medicine, but choose a shorter acting version (perhaps Metadate CD˙). If you find that that medicine doesn't work well, or it causes terrible side effects, then you would likely switch to a different category altogether—i.e. you may move over to the therapeutic amphetamines.

Let's now review some specifics about the different groups of medicines.

The Stimulants

The stimulant medicines have been around for decades. The first time a stimulant medicine was used was in 1937, when Dr. Charles Bradley of Rhode Island gave children benzedrine, and it helped their inattention, and they could do their math homework. Ritalin˙ was first marketed in 1958. There are now newer versions of these old medications—they are "new and improved." The main benefit of the newer versions of the medicines is that they last longer with one dose, and this can improve symptom control throughout the course of the day.

Within the stimulant group, as seen in Table 4, there are two main medicines:

1. Methylphenidate
2. Therapeutic Amphetamines

Methylphenidate is the generic name for Ritalin˙. As listed in Table 5 above, there are several versions which are updated forms of this medicine. They include (but are not limited to): Ritalin SR˙, Concerta˙, Ritalin LA˙, Metadate CD˙, Biphentin˙, Focalin˙, Focalin XR˙, Daytrana˙ Patch, Methylin˙, Rubifen˙.

Please note that there are certain medicines which are only available in certain countries. For example, the Daytrana skin patch is only available in the United States at the time of publication, and the medicine Biphentin is only available in Canada at this time. In general, it is fair to say that the USA has the most options for different forms of ADD medications. This relates to the fact that there are more people diagnosed and treated for ADD in the USA, and thus it is worth it for the pharmaceutical companies to develop their medicines for release in the USA.

With time, the newer options are making their way into other countries. Even if you don't have as many options for medicines in your country, you can still apply the principles of what you learn here to improve the medication treatment you receive for your son or daughter in your country.

The therapeutic amphetamines are prescription medicines which are similar to, yet significantly different than street amphetamines. They are similar in that they are in the same chemical family. They are different in that when the medicine is taken as prescribed by a doctor, they are not addictive, and do not produce a "high," like street amphetamines do.

The therapeutic amphetamines include: Vyvanse˙, Adderall˙, Adderall XR˙, Dexedrine˙, and Dexedrine Spansules˙ (see Table 5 above).

Therapeutic amphetamines work similarly in the brain to the methylphenidate medicines. That said, because they have a different chemical structure, there are some people who are going to do better with one family of medication compared to the other. This is most likely because of genetic make-up, though there may be other factors which are not yet known.

At this stage, there is no way to predict which stimulant medicine is going to work better. There is no blood test, or genetic test, or anything else of the sort. The only possible predictor is if there is a family member who has done well on one of the medicines, then it is possible that using the same one may work well for the other family member.

Getting Started With a Stimulant Medicine

When starting with a stimulant medicine, it is important to recognize some important facts about these medicines.

1) THE STIMULANTS WORK WHEN YOU TAKE THEM, AND DON'T WHEN YOU DON'T

There are many medicines in psychiatry where doses have to build up to get an effect. The stimulant medicines are not in this group. When someone takes a stimulant on Monday morning, the pill starts working in 30 to 60 minutes, and then it wears off a number of hours later (usually 8 to 12 hours for the newer medicines). The medicine is effectively out of their system by night time. If they don't take the pill on Tuesday, the medicine won't be working Tuesday, but if they take it again on Wednesday, it will work on Wednesday.

2) THE STIMULANTS MUST BE TAKEN IN THE MORNING

One of the most common side effects with the stimulant medicines is insomnia—that is trouble sleeping. If a child or teen took their pill at eight p.m., they would almost certainly be up all night long. When people take their medicine at eight a.m., the medicine generally lasts until seven or eight p.m., and then they get to sleep on time without a problem. There are some people who have this timing, but then don't fall asleep until midnight or one a.m. This is problematic insomnia—and you'll have to talk to your doctor about possibly stopping the medicine.

3) DECREASED APPETITE IS A CONCERN

The second most common side effect with the stimulant medicines is decreased appetite. It is important to have a decent breakfast before or while taking the medicine. If the medicine is taken 30 to 60 minutes before breakfast, then there is a chance that the appetite will already be gone before breakfast.

Most kids will eat breakfast well, be less hungry for lunch and snacks during the day, and then get extra hungry after the medicine wears off—and want to eat extra during the evening. They should be allowed to eat after supper if they get hungry again—just aim for healthy food choices. Occasionally I hear about parents who get upset if their child wants to eat after meal time—and, although it may not be a pattern which is common or accepted in their family, I encourage it in the case of ADD medication.

If appetite suppression carries on, there is a chance of losing weight. Weight loss can be a concern—particularly for the kids or teens who are thin to begin with. If this is the case, monitor this closely with the doctor.

4) WATCH FOR GROWTH SLOWING

Research has looked at the slowing of growth over the decades of stimulant medicine usage. At this time, the best research suggests that approximately two to three percent of kids who take stimulant medicines will have some slowing of growth. It is not clear what the mechanism of this growth slowing is. It also seems as if the slowed growth is in the range of one inch below the expected height.

While taking stimulant medicines, it is important to have the doctor monitor height and weight on a growth chart to make sure that there is not a drop-off in height which is a concern.

5) TICS

In a small percentage of people, there is a chance of bringing out tics or twitches from the medication. There is no scientific evidence of these medicines causing tics, rather, that they bring out tics in people who are prone to them.

When reviewing tics, it's important to know that there are *motor* tics and *voca*l tics.

Motor tics include muscle movements. These would include: excessive blinking, a mouth movement, a neck tic, or other variations. There are some "complex" tics meaning that they involve more than one muscle group—i.e. tics such as repeatedly drumming on things or making a throwing gesture with the arm.

Vocal tics include sounds. They can be yelps and "whoops," or even things like sniffing, snorting, or repetitive throat clearing.

When stimulant medicines bring out tics, often they are mild, and they stop when the medicine is stopped. On occasion, however, the tics become quite problematic, and interfere with functioning.

If tics are a concern, talk to your doctor. Your doctor may recommend stopping the medication, continuing and monitoring the tics, or even continuing with the medicine, and adding a second medicine to deal with the tics. When making this decision, it will be important to remember the "risk-benefit ratio." How much are the medicines helping, and what are the risks if you stop the ADD medication.

6) MOOD SYMPTOMS

Although relatively rare, it is possible to get mood side effects from stimulant medicines. These may be excessive sadness, significant irritability or agitation, or even excited or manic behavior. If these are a concern, talk to your doctor right away.

7) FLATTENING OF PERSONALITY

This is often an unspoken concern of many parents and, to be sure, of many teens with ADD. They may be interested in a medicine to help with ADD, but they don't want their personality changed. They always know someone who knows someone who "turned into a robot" when taking ADD medications.

In reality, this is a relatively rare side effect. When it does happen, I treat it as a real side effect—as concerning as serious insomnia or some other physical side effect.

The goal when treating ADD with medication is to treat the ADD symptoms so that your child can be himself/herself without the ADD symptoms getting in the way. The medicine will treat the inattention, hyperactivity and impulsivity but it is important that it doesn't block the spontaneity. There is a subtle yet important difference between impulsivity and spontaneity. I always reassure parents and kids/teens that if this side effect becomes an issue, I will help them by either changing the medication dose, or changing the medication altogether.

8) MEDICATION HOLIDAYS?

Because the stimulants can be taken on some days and not others, you may wonder about not giving the medication on weekends, or school breaks. In fact, the experts in ADD recommended for many years just to treat ADD during the school week—because the medicine was needed to help with school.

In recent years, research has shown that ADD has a big impact on social, emotional and psychological factors as well, and it is important to treat for these. In other words, if we help kids to focus better in school, yet they are doing terribly socially and emotionally, we aren't helping them for the long term. As such, the current recommendations are to take medication seven days per week, throughout the year.

There are some families who decide to stop the medication during the school breaks and summer breaks. This can be helpful in certain circumstances— i.e. if there is significant weight loss and your son needs to be able to gain a few pounds during the summer, for example. Of course, review these issues with your doctor.

9) ARE STIMULANT MEDICINES ADDICTIVE?

This has been a big concern for parents for many years. Here is the short answer: when stimulants for ADD are taken as prescribed, there is no risk of people becoming addicted to them.

You'll recall that one of the risks of untreated ADD is that people can be prone to drug and alcohol addictions. This is often caused by the fact that they "self medicate" with the drugs and alcohol to control their irritability, hyperactivity, or inattention. There have been several studies done which have followed young people who were taking Ritalin daily and monitored them from childhood to adolescence. When looking at reviews of these studies (in "meta-analyses," which are studies which group different studies together so that one may draw common conclusions from other studies), they generally show a dramatic lowering of future drug and alcohol problems when kids take medicines for ADD.

The tricky part of this discussion is that ADD medications can be abused, misused or *diverted.*

Abuse of the medicines refers to the fact that they are taken to get a high. Misuse means they are taken in a way that they are not intended for—i.e. a college student has a prescription for an ADD medication, but takes extra the night before an exam so that he can stay up all night to study.

Diversion refers to the medicine being diverted to someone else— for a different person and a different purpose than it was prescribed for. For example, if someone sells their prescription to a friend, so that friend can get high, or even study—that is diversion.

When reviewing abuse, the medicines can be abused if they are taken in a way which is different from the intention of the prescription. For example, the short acting forms of the stimulants—i.e. Ritalin, Dexedrine, or Adderall Immediate Release—can be abused. When these pills are crushed up, they can be snorted and then they can produce a high. Although this may seem absurd or scary for parents to know—it is important to be aware of this—so you are fully informed. In the Toronto area, short acting 10 mg Ritalin® pills have a street value of five dollars. Certain drug dealers will sell Ritalin® for teens to get high. There will be teens who try to get prescriptions for short acting ADD medications so that they can either abuse the drugs themselves, or sell them to others to earn money—possibly so that they can buy different drugs.

This issue has been helped significantly by the newer, long acting medicines. The long acting medicines are much less likely to be abused, because they have delayed release mechanisms in them which prevent rapid absorption—rapid absorption is needed to produce a high. If you are concerned about this, ask your doctor and he can review the issue with you, while reviewing the best treatment for your child or teen.

When it comes to misuse or diversion, these are issues which must be monitored. Stimulant medicines are generally treated as "controlled substances" and most states have controls in place to monitor how doctors prescribe these. Often times, doctors cannot renew a prescription by phone for this group of medicines. Doctors will also become concerned if you phone and ask for a new prescription two days after you just got one (even if you legitimately lost it) because this could mean that you are misusing the pills.

The First Prodrug for ADD

The newer generation of stimulant medicines consists of the old, effective medications (which are short acting) and putting them into higher tech pills which deliver the medicine over the course of the day with only one dose. For example, Ritalin® needs to be taken at eight a.m., noon and four p.m. to get a full day of symptom control. However, the newer pill Concerta® has the same active ingredient, but it releases the medicine in a steady fashion over the course of the day after one dose in the morning.

Most of the newer medicines just use a high tech delivery system to deliver the medicine—i.e. a delayed release bead (like Adderall XR®), or a modified capsule to deliver the medicine more steadily through the day (like Concerta®). In 2007, a new medicine came to market in the US which had a completely different approach. It is called Vyvanse®.

Vyvanse® is a *prodrug*. This means that the medicine is not active until an enzyme in the body acts on it. The medicine is the active ingredient dextroamphetamine (which is the same as Dexedrine, and very similar to Adderall), which is chemically bonded to lysine, an amino acid (or protein building block). The medicine is rapidly absorbed by the stomach, but it is not active in the brain until an enzyme in the body breaks the bond between the dextroamphetamine and the lysine. This causes a gradual release of the medicine throughout the day, and permits a very reliable absorption.

Vyvanse® has been found to last up to 13 hours in kids, whereas the other stimulants only last 12 hours. In my initial experience with it (it came to Canada in 2010), I find that it can be quite smooth in its onset and offset, and this can lead to good results. Vyvanse® is also much less abusable than the other stimulants, because it takes time for the body to convert it to active medicine—if someone tried to snort it, they wouldn't get a rapid high.

Vyvanse is mentioned because it is currently the only prodrug for ADD, and it seems to have unique features. You can talk to your doctor about it if you have questions.

Getting Started with the Non-Stimulant Medicines

When it comes to the non-stimulant medicines, these are newer to the scene of treating ADD. There are many doctors who are used to the stimulant medicines, and they feel more comfortable using them to treat ADD. When it comes down to it, the two main non-stimulants, Strattera® and Intuniv®, are both "first line" for ADD. This means that they have been approved by the FDA in the US for the treatment of ADD. That said, there are many doctors who may not choose to use them as their first choice. There is a difference between "first line" and "first choice." Even though a medicine is first line, a doctor may not choose to use it first. This often depends on the doctor's previous experiences, as well as his knowledge of the medicine. Of course this is completely reasonable, however there are some doctors who will never use a certain medicine for ADD (whether they avoid non-stimulants, or even amphetamines). Since not everyone responds equally to the different medicines, it is important that the new options be used when necessary, and that your son or daughter has the opportunity to try a medication which may help them.

The non-stimulants work differently than the stimulants. Strattera® has to be taken daily, and it will take approximately four to six weeks to work. When it does work, it will work around the clock, meaning it will work in the early morning, through the day, and into the evening as well. Because Strattera has to be taken daily, it cannot be stopped on weekends, or it will lose its effect. Intuniv® has to be taken daily as well. It will start working more quickly than Strattera, and its benefits may wear off by night time, or in some individuals, it may last until the next morning.

One of the main benefits of the non-stimulants is that they are not abusable at all. There is no chance that anyone can get high from these medicines. Consequently, they don't have a street value. Because of this fact, these medicines are not "controlled substances." This means that pharmacies and doctors do not have the same controls imposed on them. Prescriptions can be called in on the phone and they can be repeated much more easily.

Information about Strattera®

Strattera® works by primarily blocking the re-uptake of norepinephrine (this means that it boosts the amount of norepinephrine—in the manner described earlier).

Its most common side effects are sleepiness and nausea. Your doctor will generally calculate the dose based on your child's weight. The dose administered will start low for several days, then it will be raised to a middle dose, and then to a starting dose within two to four weeks. The gradual increase in the dose will help your child's body get used to the side effects of the medication—i.e. nausea and fatigue in particular. Some doctors will increase the dose more quickly than described above. If your doctor does this, and your child is getting too many side effects, ask for a more gradual increase.

Strattera® has the benefit of not causing or worsening tics. If someone has a tic disorder, or has worsened tics from a stimulant medicine, then Strattera is a good option to consider.

Additionally, Strattera® has data indicating that it helps to improve anxiety when it is present with ADD. So if your child has ADD plus an Anxiety disorder, your doctor may suggest Strattera as an option—because Strattera can be one medicine which treats both groups of symptoms.

Also, because Strattera® has no abuse potential, some doctors may choose it if your teen has a drug or alcohol problem. When Strattera® is used, there is no chance that your teen could try to abuse the ADD medicine, or even try to sell it or trade it for other drugs. And if there is a family member with a drug or alcohol problem, the doctor may suggest Strattera® as well, to help to reduce the chance of misuse or abuse.

When Strattera® was being researched, there was one case of liver toxicity. This means that the individual's liver stopped working properly due to the Strattera®. When the medicine was stopped, this reaction went away. The person experienced jaundice (i.e. skin turning yellow), itchy skin, and multiple other symptoms and the lab work was very abnormal. While there is a warning on Strattera® because of this, it is extremely rare—and after millions of prescriptions have been written worldwide, there is still just one case reported. There is no need for regular blood work to monitor for liver functions. Rather, call your doctor if your child is feeling very sick, or looking very sick, particularly if they are jaundiced (i.e. having yellow skin when you look at their skin in the sunlight).

Strattera® was also found to have a higher rate of suicidal ideas in kids and teens when compared to placebo. The rate of Strattera® causing suicidal ideas is 0.4 percent—meaning four kids or teens per thousand treated. While this is a very low rate, it is significant because suicidal ideas constitute such a serious side effect. If your doctor is prescribing Strattera®, it is important that the doctor have a discussion about safety regarding suicidal ideas before starting the medicine.

The suicidal ideas generally come in the first weeks or months of treatment. In general, this side effect is less of a concern in younger kids, and more of a concern in teenagers. With teens, it's important for the doctor to review a safety plan and a risk assessment for suicidal ideas before starting the medicine. The suicidal ideas were not found to be a symptom related to Strattera® in adults who take it for ADD. Obviously this is an important area for you to talk to your doctor about.

Information About Intuniv®

Intuniv® is a non-stimulant for ADD which works in a different way than the other ADD medications. It is an "alpha agonist." This means that it works on different receptors in the neuron (or brain cell). When it does its work, it is calming, it helps with hyperactivity/impulsivity, and it also helps with concentration. The most common side effect with Intuniv® is sedation (sleepiness). It is derived from an old high blood pressure pill, so it can lower heart rate and blood pressure slightly. If this becomes a problematic side effect, your child could get dizzy or even faint. Your doctor should monitor heart rate and blood pressure while your child is taking this medicine. Intuniv® is generally taken in the morning, and lasts for up to 24 hours.

Because Intuniv® has an impact on kid's blood pressure (i.e. it can drop it slightly), it is important for your child or teen to not stop this medicine abruptly. If you would like to stop this medicine, it is important to talk to your doctor about gradually tapering the medication.

What about Combinations of Medicines?

There are times that doctors may suggest taking more than one ADD medicine to get a good effect.

Taking Two Stimulants:

Generally, people won't take two different stimulants. Someone may take a long acting stimulant and then "top it up" with a short acting form of the same medicine at the end of the day (i.e. taking 54 mg Concerta® in the morning, and then taking short acting Ritalin® 10 mg at five p.m.).

Taking a Stimulant and a Non-Stimulant:

There are times that doctors will add a non-stimulant to a stimulant. For example, being on Vyvanse® for the daytime ADD symptom control, and then taking Intuniv® to help with sleep. Or taking Adderall XR® during the daytime, and Strattera® as well, so that it can help to boost the anti-ADD effects of the medicine.

The stimulants and non-stimulants work differently, so it can be okay to use them together. Often times, you need to have a doctor with more expertise in ADD to feel comfortable with doing this.

Warnings on ADD Medicines

Any medication can have rare but serious side effects. In recent years, there have been warnings about the ADD medications. This section will provide an overview of these warnings, and it is recommended that you talk to your doctor or read more online if you want more specific information about these medications. These warnings refer to all of the stimulant medicines and the non-stimulant Strattera®. The warnings do not apply to Intuniv®.

1) **CARDIOVASCULAR SIDE EFFECTS:** All of the ADD medications (except for Intuniv®) raise the heart rate and blood pressure slightly. This is so little that for a healthy individual, it would have no impact. However, there are risk factors which have an impact on the cardiovascular side effects. If your child

has a structural heart abnormality (i.e. a "hole in the heart"), or irregular heartbeats, talk to the doctor about seeing a pediatric heart specialist before taking the medicines.

If your child cannot run up stairs or exercise appropriately, then talk to the doctor. If there have been any cardiac deaths in your family members— under the age of 50—this can indicate a genetic risk for irregular heartbeats or heart problems. The biggest risk for the cardiovascular side effects is sudden death. Although this has been a concern, a recent review of the research by Harvard psychiatrists found that the rate of cardiac death of children on ADD medications was equal to the rate of cardiac death in children who were not on ADD medications[2], suggesting that there is no increased risk.

Do you need an EKG?

After the concerns were raised about cardiovascular side effects, there were doctors and medical organizations who recommended routine EKGs being done on each person before they started taking a stimulant medication. Further review of the research has suggested that this is not necessary. If you are concerned about these issues, you can certainly ask your child's doctor about getting an EKG.

There is an excellent review paper on this issue, written jointly by Canadian Pediatricians, Child Psychiatrists, and Cardiologists. It provides an excellent review of the science about ADD medications, EKGs and cardiac deaths. If you are interested in reading more about this, you can access this paper online via the link in the footnote below.[3]

---

2   Wilens et al. "Stimulants and sudden death: what is a physician to do?" Pediatrics. 2006 Sep; 118(3): 1215-9

3   http://www.cacap-acpea.org/files/2009%20November%20cardiac%20risk.pdf

2) **PSYCHIATRIC SIDE EFFECTS:** The ADD medications can cause psychiatric side effects, including psychosis and agitation (this again refers to the stimulants and Strattera®, and not Intuniv®).

Psychosis refers to being out of touch with reality in some way—i.e. hallucinations and delusions. Hallucinations are abnormal sensory perceptions (i.e. seeing things that aren't there, hearing voices, etc.). Delusions are fixed false beliefs—i.e. becoming paranoid when there is no evidence that it is based on facts.

Psychosis is quite a rare side effect of the ADD medications, but it is a serious one. If this happens, call the doctor immediately, and you can consider going to the Emergency Room (ER) if it is after hours.

Agitation refers to your child or teen becoming agitated, restless, or excessively irritable. If it becomes severe, it can lead to significant concerns or issues. If this happens, again, call the doctor or consider going to the ER if needed.

How Long Does My Child Need To Take ADD Medications?

Before wrapping up this chapter, I wanted to include a question that most parents ask as they are starting ADD medications. It is hard enough to decide to take the medications—and it becomes even harder if you think that you are putting your son or daughter on medication for years or for the rest of his/her life.

When parents, kids and teens are considering medication for ADD, I like to break the treatment down into short term, medium term and long term.

In the short term, we take one to three months to find the right medicine, adjust dosing, deal with side effects, and see if it even works. If we can find a medicine that works well, and is free of side effects (or has minimal, manageable side effects), then it is worth carrying on with the medicine.

In the medium term, it is worth taking the medicine for this school year, and maybe next. This is a judgement call to be made with your doctor.

In the longer term, I generally suggest that every one or two years that you should start the school year with the medication, and then after one month or so, stop it and see how things go. You can either tell the teacher that you are doing an experiment, or you may decide not to tell the teacher.

If your child has developed good coping skills, and improved, he may do well without the medication. If he struggles, then he needs the medicine again. If he does well without the medication, then you still need to actively monitor his functioning, because if he develops symptoms of concern again, then he may need to restart the medicine (think of the analogy of an adult with high blood pressure—if the adult gets it under control with diet and exercise, and then it goes out of control again, the doctor will want to start the medicines to protect against any long term risks).

Knowing what you already know about the duration of ADD—many kids have it into adolescents, and about 30 to 40 percent of them outgrow ADD by adult life—there is therefore a majority of people who still have ADD as an adult. The question is: will your child have to take medicine into the adult years?

There are some people who take medicine for years—because their functioning and quality of life is that much better with it (and their side effects are minimal or manageable). That said, there are some adults who develop great coping skills and structure in their lives, and they may choose not to use medication.

As a teen grows, hopefully he develops his passions and goes into an area of study or a profession which is exciting and stimulating to him. If he does, then it will be much easier for him to focus, and he may not need medication to help. That said, even if he loves being a computer programmer, or graphic designer, he will still have to pay bills, file taxes and get along in his relationships. If these other areas become a concern, then it is worth looking at medication as well.

CHAPTER 8

Step 6: Alternative Treatments for ADD

a s we progress with the Attention Difference Disorder System for ADD, the next step to consider is the alternative treatments for ADD.

Many people use alternative treatments—yet they often don't talk to their doctor about it. Recent research documented that 66 percent of parents admit to using some sort of alternative treatment for their ADD child, yet only 11 percent have told their doctor about it.

Why don't people tell their doctor if they use alternatives? The reason is simple—most doctors are not open to the alternatives, and then they can be judgmental about your decisions. When that happens, it can be even harder for you—as a parent who is working hard to help your child, and often fighting "against the current."

The simple solution to this situation is better knowledge about the alternative treatments—both for parents and for doctors. This chapter will start that journey for you.

It is my belief that every treatment plan for ADD should at least consider, if not implement, some aspect of alternative treatment.

Alternative vs. Complementary Treatments

While I've named this chapter "alternative treatments," I really mean complementary. What's the difference?

The term alternative treatment refers to treatments that are used *instead of* standard medical care. If you were doing purely alternative treatments, you would avoid standard medical care for ADD, which includes multimodal treatment—including medication, parenting support, academic strategies, therapy, etc. This would leave out significantly helpful and well researched treatments which can help ADD.

Complementary treatments refer to treatments which are done *in addition to* standard medical care. I strongly advocate this approach when adding newer, so called "alternative treatments." This means that in addition to using parenting strategies and academic strategies, you are using neurofeedback. Or in addition to taking medication, you are modifying the diet, or taking supplements such as Omega 3 fatty acids.

If I mean complementary treatments, why did I call the chapter "alternative treatments"? This relates to the fact that when I talk to parents, most parents use the term "alternative." It's my goal in this book to support you in where you are, therefore I've named the chapter "alternatives" and I will be using that term throughout the chapter. However, remember that I am encouraging a complementary approach.

Remember—treatment of ADD is a marathon not a sprint.

While working on your long term ADD marathon, you may try different strategies along the way. If something works, then stick with it. If it doesn't, then move on and try something different.

Research behind Alternative Treatments for ADD

One of the main reasons that doctors are hesitant about alternatives for ADD relates to the fact that there is a lot less research done on alternatives than there is for the standard treatments for ADD. When research is done for the alternative treatments, doctors don't often know about it, and they often criticize the research that has been done.

The standard thinking about research methods is that the best studies are randomized, double blind, placebo controlled trials. These trials are designed to compare an active treatment vs. a placebo treatment. The design is set up so that there will be little bias, so that the researchers can really tell if the active treatment works.

For example, if people were allowed to choose if they wanted to take a medication, or if they wanted to take a placebo at the start of the study—and they knew which one they got—then the results of each assessment would be significantly influenced by their knowledge.

However, if the study is randomized, the people can't choose which treatment they get. In addition if it is blind, they don't know which one they got. It follows then that when they are giving feedback about how their treatment is doing at each visit in the research study, they are giving accurate accounts of what has been happening without any bias based on their beliefs about their treatments.

The problem with research in alternative treatments is that it is often very hard to design a study to meet the criteria of a randomized, double blind, placebo controlled trial. A clear example is homeopathy. Homeopathic treatment must be individualized. That means that each person would take different remedies, even if they had the same medical diagnosis of ADD. There is no way to blind a research study for classical homeopathy. Other treatments have attempted to have more scientifically rigorous designs to show that the treatments work, yet the scientific and medical community is quick to disregard these as flawed studies.

One of the other big issues with research into alternative treatments relates to the funding of this research. Research trials are very costly. When it comes to medication, there are pharmaceutical companies who invest heavily in the research necessary to bring a medicine to market—and thus they fund research that could benefit them ultimately. They know that they could earn a profit later from a patented medicine resulting from that research. The medicines are patented for a number of years, and no one else is allowed to make that medicine—allowing the company time to recuperate their investment and earn a profit. When it comes to alternative treatments, there are few companies who are able to invest in the research, and if they do, often a competitor can just market the same product right away and take away their ability to profit—because there is no patent. So, less research is done into alternative treatments overall.

Why am I willing to be open to alternative treatments, even if there are design problems in the studies, and not enough research being done?

The answer is simple. It's because that is what my patients are doing. By listening to my patients, I realized that this is what they were doing. It is important to me to support my patients in their treatment—even if I initially wasn't certain about the research on the alternative treatments.

What I've done, is I've looked up the research on the different alternative treatments which people commonly use and I use this information to have open discussions about alternatives with my patients.

I'll summarize that research in the following sections.

Guiding Principles in Choosing Alternatives

1) PRINCIPLE 1: THE LEVEL OF EVIDENCE NEEDED DEPENDS ON THE TREATMENT

When looking at any medical treatment, it is important to look at the level of evidence which is needed based on the nature of the treatment. For example, if you were going to consider taking chemotherapy for cancer, you need more information to make an informed decision than if you were going to consider taking a multivitamin in the morning. While this example demonstrates an extreme difference, it is important to remember this principle. If an alternative treatment will cost five thousand dollars, and take two nights per week for four months, you will likely want more evidence that it will work, compared to taking a vitamin in the morning.

2) PRINCIPLE 2: LOOK FOR REAL RESEARCH

When looking at the evidence for an alternative treatment, it is important to look for actual research, not just testimonials or case studies. When people are marketing a treatment, they can often use testimonials. The testimonial often consists of a happy mother's picture saying that this treatment has made all of the difference for her ADD son. These types of testimonials are designed to pull on your heart strings to get you to buy their product. It is best to look for scientific research which has been published in a scientific journal. It is best if the journal is "peer reviewed," meaning that other doctors/scientists reviewed the studies to ensure that there was a standard of research met. When looking at research, take a close look at the sample that was studied. If you have an eight year old girl with ADD, and you find that the research was done on teenage boys with ADD—it is hard to know if the treatment will work with your daughter.

3) PRINCIPLE 3: BE CAREFUL WITH HERBS

If you are considering taking herbal treatments, then be careful about possible psycho-active actions of these medicines. This refers to the fact that the herbal treatments can have an impact on the thoughts and moods of those who take them. They can also have drug interactions. Therefore, if your son or daughter has to take medication for a medical condition, be sure to check regarding the safety of herbal treatments. This is not meant to say that all herbal treatments are a problem—far from it. This is intended to remind you that just because something is "natural" doesn't mean it isn't harmless. Remember, marijuana, psilocybin mushrooms (i.e. magic mushrooms), and cyanide are all natural!

4) PRINCIPLE 4: GET PROFESSIONAL HELP

If you are having tax problems, you get an accountant. If you are having tooth pain, you see a dentist. If you have ADD, you'll likely see a psychiatrist, psychologist or pediatrician. If you want to start alternative or complementary treatment, it is worth seeing an expert in that field to provide guidance and expertise. Look in your community for people with professional training, and who have experience with ADD. You can ask at a parent support group—someone may know of a great doctor to help you. Often times, people will start with a Naturopathic Doctor.

One caution about finding a professional—make sure that the philosophy of the doctor matches your philosophy. For example, there are some "alternative medicine doctors" who have extremely negative views of ADD, as well as the medical profession as a whole. If you are going to see an alternative professional, ensure that their philosophy is compatible with yours, and hopefully your doctor's. One specific thing to consider is: if you decide to use medication, will this alternative medicine professional still provide help and work with you? Or will they judge you and make you feel bad for trying it? These are important questions to ask before investing your time and money in a treatment professional.

5) PRINCIPLE 5: REMEMBER THAT DELAYING A PROVEN ADD TREATMENT CAN BE A RISK

As we discussed in Step 5, Medications for ADD, there are many factors to consider when deciding on ADD medication. One of those factors is the severity of the ADD. If the severity is moderate to high, and if the impairment is moderate to high, then if you take a long time to find an effective treatment, you are potentially at risk of problems developing. I am not suggesting that it is not worth trying alternatives. This chapter is intended to help you to find alternatives which may help you. Rather, this principle is meant to help you to avoid a situation which I see all too often in my office. The following illustrative example will help you to understand.

Several years ago, I saw two new patients in my office one morning. Let's call them *Case 1* and *Case 2*.

Case 1: The first new patient I saw that morning was a seven year old boy who was diagnosed with ADD. The symptoms were moderate, and the parents were very caring, concerned and educated. They were reluctant to try medication. After I completed my assessment, the family asked a lot of questions, and we discussed my suggestions about the treatment options for their son. When I suggested a trial of medication, they said that they wanted to hold off, because they were about to try some alternative treatments—specifically diet for ADD. They said they didn't want medication now, and if that was what I was recommending, then they thought they didn't need to come back and see me again. As a child psychiatrist in a community with a severe shortage of child psychiatrists, I just agreed with them. If they wanted to work with other professionals, in that case I had no concerns with that. (I never saw the patient again).

Case 2: Ten minutes after finishing that consultation, I met another family. Mom and Dad were both present for the appointment, with a 15 year old girl who clearly didn't want to be in my office. When I started getting the story, what I learned was that when "Alice" was eight years old, she was diagnosed with ADD. The doctor who diagnosed ADD recommended medication, but the parents were reluctant and wanted to try alternative treatment. They weren't sure if they agreed with the diagnosis of ADD, and they weren't convinced about the need for medication. They weren't sure that they even agreed with the idea of medicating a child for "behavior."

Alice's parents went to a Naturopathic Doctor, and were instructed to give their daughter certain supplements, and to eliminate many foods from her diet. When I asked, they didn't recall all of the details of the supplements or the diet change. What they did recall was that the diet was hard to maintain—it eliminated wheat, dairy, sugar, eggs, etc. The parents said that they worked hard at this treatment regimen for about three months. They think it may have helped, but they weren't sure. Then, life got busy, the treatment was costly, and they just let it go. Alice went for seven years without any treatment for ADD (alternative or medical), and without any medical assessments and follow up for her ADD.

When the parents were sitting in my office, they described that they were so concerned about how terribly things had turned out. Their daughter was skipping school so much, that she could be expelled. She was smoking marijuana daily, and they thought she was sexually active. She had been charged by police for shoplifting and seemed to show no remorse. She was so defiant at home that the parents felt she was completely out of control. The parents literally asked me to prescribe any medication that I thought would help. They were feeling desperate that their daughter was slipping away from them and they had to act now or it would be too late. I worked with the parents and Alice to help them improve the situation.

As I reflected on what happened that morning, I came to some important conclusions. It was clear to me that Case 1 was a similar story as was Case 2 when she was first diagnosed. The parents in Case 1 wanted to pursue alternatives, and they were not going to follow up with me; that likely meant that they would not get ongoing assessment and support for ADD. Case 2 had a lot of the long term risks of untreated ADD (though they don't always manifest so completely). I felt that the doctor who initially saw Alice did her a disservice by not asking her to come back in three months, to see how she was doing. By not supporting the parents' exploration into alternatives, the doctor ended up inadvertently supporting a significant downward turn for Alice over seven years. To be clear, I am not blaming the doctor, nor am I blaming the parents or Alice. What I did learn was that it is important to provide ongoing follow up, to be open to alternative treatments, and to support a family with its needs—educationally (i.e. to learn more about ADD), emotionally, and treatment needs at their own pace.

Therefore, when I recommend that you consider the fact that delaying proven treatments can be a risk, realize that I mean both for the short term and the long term. On the one hand, if the school principle says that if the misbehavior doesn't improve by Friday, then he will be expelled—he needs immediate treatment. On the other hand, if the situation is like Alice's described above, then there is a longer term risk because the treatment was delayed for too long.

In this chapter, we will cover seven types of alternative treatments for ADD, including:

1. Diet Change for ADD
2. Omega 3 Fatty Acids
3. Homeopathy for ADD
4. Herbal Treatments/Supplements
5. Neurofeedback for ADD
6. Cerebellar Treatments
7. Software Working Memory Training

Therapy #1: Diet Change for ADD

Diet change for ADD has been around for decades. There have been numerous research attempts to prove a connection between diet and ADD, and numerous research attempts to prove that there is no connection. The National Institutes of Mental Health (in the USA) held a consensus meeting in the 1980s to determine that there was no benefit to diet changes for ADD.

The Feingold Diet has been around for approximately three decades. They claim great results for ADD, as well as many other conditions such as Autism, Dyslexia, Irritable Bowel Syndrome, Seizures and more.[1] We will review the Feingold diet in more detail shortly.

There have been two medical research studies published in the recent past which have been quite instructive with respect to ADD and diet.

The first was a paper published in the prestigious medical journal, *The Lancet* in November 2007.[2] This study took children from the community in two age ranges—either three years old, or eight to nine years old. They enrolled these children in the study, and initially all food dyes and preservatives were removed from their diet. This was done before the study commenced (this was called a "washout" period). Then the researchers gave the kids juice to drink; the juice either contained a placebo, or food dyes and preservatives. The children were studied over a six week period, and the researchers found when the children were taking the food dyes and preservatives, that the rate of ADD symptoms was higher than when they weren't. This research suggests that the food dyes and preservatives, which are very common in the western diet, can in fact be contributing to ADD symptoms. Please note that the study did not prove that food additives cause ADD. The study also doesn't prove that if you stop food additives that ADD will be gone.

---

1   http://www.feingold.org/ Accessed September, 2010

2   *The Lancet* (2007) McCann, D et al: "Food Additives and hyperactive behaviour in 3 year-old and 8/9 year-old children in the community: a randomised, double-blinded, placebo-controlled trial"; Volume 370, p 1560-1567

This study is quite important for many reasons. Firstly, it was published in a very well regarded medical journal. This means that even the most skeptical doctors will take note of its findings. Secondly, it shows a connection between food dyes and preservatives and children's ADD symptoms. This study has taken the attention of many medical organizations, and some are considering adding the recommendation of "removing food additives from the diet" to their ADD treatment guidelines.

How does this apply to you? It may be reasonable to consider cutting out the unnecessary chemicals in your child's diet. Consider a trial of eliminating food dyes and preservatives.

The second study which is quite important regarding ADD and diet came out of Europe in 2009. This study was called "A Randomised Controlled Trial into the Effects of Food."[3] In this study, the researchers enrolled 27 kids with a mean age of six years old (80 percent of them were boys). They were monitored on their own diet for two weeks, and then they were randomized to either a "few foods diet," or their regular diet for a period of six weeks. The researchers monitored their ADD symptoms and behavior.

The "few foods diet" is an elimination diet which consisted of 10 foods. It included only rice, turkey, lamb, vegetables, fruits, margarine, vegetable oil, tea, pear juice and water.

At the end of the trial, the researchers found that the number of clinical responders in the few foods diet group was 73 percent vs. 0 percent in the placebo group. There was also a reduction in the measured oppositional defiant disorder in the diet group as well.

This study was well designed, and showed a significant improvement with ADD and ODD symptoms in six year olds eating a few foods diet.

What does this mean for you?

3   Eur Child Adolesc Psychiatry (2009) 18: 12-19; Pelsser, et al: "A randomised controlled trial into the effects of food on ADHD."

This may mean that an elimination diet could be helpful. Certainly in this study, there were significant and measurable results from this diet change.

In my experience, if parents are going to start an elimination diet, it is best to try it when children are younger. When kids are in the six to eight year old range, it is easier to control what they are eating, and to "enforce" the elimination diet. During the teen years, it is much harder to get teens to follow an elimination diet.

The Feingold Diet

This diet was mentioned briefly earlier. Although I haven't found research which is as strong as the studies described above, I think it is important to review, as many parents can use this as a starting point. The Feingold website has a lot of information, and can be found here: *www.feingold.org*

The Feingold diet is essentially an elimination diet. There are two main phases:

1) Eliminate food with specific additives and chemicals (and observe behavior/improvement); then

2) Gradually re-introduce foods and evaluate the symptoms.

One of the main principles of the Feingold diet is to avoid foods with the chemical "salicylates." There are both synthetic salicylates, and natural salicylates. The synthetic salicylates generally contain the letters "sal" or "salicylate" in them—for example salicylic acid. The natural salicylates include foods like: almonds, cucumber, peaches, raisins, etc. You can find a comprehensive list on the Feingold website.

The Feingold diet also encourages you to avoid other additives such as: synthetic colorings, artificial flavors, artificial preservatives and all artificial sweeteners.

Although there may not be enough research to fully endorse the Feingold diet, in my opinion, it is a good place for many families to start. Committing to a full Feingold diet can be challenging for many families—especially if there are more kids in the family than just your ADD child.

If it is hard to commit to a full Feingold diet, I recommend considering a modified Feingold, where you just eliminate food additives and dyes and monitor the response. This is in line with the first research study mentioned above. While there isn't a strong scientific base for this recommendation, there is no harm in eating a more healthy diet with few chemicals. And it may help.

As a final suggestion for diet—it is a good idea to monitor the intake of simple sugars and simple carbohydrates. This will help to avoid "sugar crashes." While many people assert that sugar causes ADD symptoms, there is no reliable research to prove that. However, in my experience, there are some kids who respond terribly to sugar, and they do much better when their parents cut it out of their diet.

Avoid Sugar Crashes

When it comes to having a snack, if someone were to have a can of soda (full of sugar) and a candy bar, they have just given themselves a very high dose of simple sugar. As the ingested soda and candy bar are absorbed, the amount of sugar in their blood stream rises quickly. Their body then senses the increase in blood sugar, and the pancreas releases insulin to control the blood sugar level. When the insulin starts to work, the blood sugar drops quickly, because the sugar which was ingested was a "simple" sugar, meaning that it was quickly absorbed, causing it to drop off rapidly.

Through the thousands of years of our body's evolution, our pancreas didn't develop to work on simple sugars like the ones found in sodas and candy bars. Our pancreas was designed to secrete insulin to match complex carbohydrates like whole wheats, brown rices, and non-processed foods. The insulin in the body is slower to start working (compared to how quickly sugar is absorbed from the "snack"), and it is slower to stop working. When the insulin is working, and the blood sugar starts to drop, then the insulin can't shut off right away, even though the simple sugar is gone.

What results is a period of relative low blood sugar. It is not a low blood sugar that can lead to the need to seek medical care (as can happen with an insulin dependent diabetic), but it is low blood sugar which can cause physical symptoms (like shaky hands, headaches, etc.), and emotional symptoms (like moodiness, irritability and anger). Many adults, who go through this, describe that when they have their sugary snacks, they have 90 minutes until they feel irritable, and then they have another sugary snack to try to make it through another 90 minutes.

To avoid this possible impact on your ADD child, consider cutting out foods with simple sugar. This includes candy, soda, etc., as well as foods with simple carbohydrates like white bread, white rice, etc. Instead, choose foods with complex carbohydrates—like whole wheat bread and brown rice. And adding protein can be helpful as well. Protein can help to stabilize blood sugar levels—particularly when taken with a carbohydrate.

Takeaways for Diet Change and ADD

- A well designed study showed that food additives can cause symptoms similar to ADD.
- A well designed study showed that an elimination diet (called the "few foods" diet) helped six year olds with ADD.
- The Feingold diet may be a good place to start for many families, either as a full Feingold elimination diet, or as a partial or modified Feingold.
- Do your best to avoid "sugar crashes" by avoiding refined sugars and having more protein for snacks.

Therapy #2: Omega 3 Fatty Acids

Omega 3 fatty acids are an "essential" nutrient. This means that our body doesn't produce them, and they have to be taken in by our diet.

To understand how Omega 3s work, it's important to understand that 60 percent of our brains are made up of fat. The fat in our brains is used to make the linings that cover the nerve wiring from one cell to another. And Omega 3 fatty acids play a role in those linings.

There are actually two essential fatty acids: Omega 3 fatty acids and Omega 6 fatty acids. For optimal health, the ratio between Omega 6s and Omega 3s should be 1:1. However, in a typical western diet, the ratio can be as high as 20:1 or 40:1! This means that there are far more Omega 6s than 3s in the typical western diet. This relates to the fact that Omega 6s are commonly found in vegetable oils (which are regularly consumed in a western diet), whereas Omega 3s are predominantly found in fish (which are not regularly consumed in a western diet). When the ratio of Omega 6 to Omega 3 is so far off, this can produce some "strain" on the individual. Theoretically, this can lead to the issues of ADD, learning disabilities, and potentially even mood disorders. Research is being done which is starting to show that Omega 3s can help in each of these conditions.

A recent published study was a randomized trial of Omega 3 fatty acids in ADD.[4] This study examined the effect of supplementing Omega 3 and omega 6 fatty acids in 75 kids and teens with ADD (aged eight to 18 years). 85 percent of the subjects were male. After three months of treatment, the majority of kids and teens did not respond to the Omega 3/6 supplementation, but 26 percent did respond, with a 25 percent reduction of symptoms. After six months, the rate went up to 46 percent who responded. To be clear, the response rate of 25 percent reduction of symptoms is not large; however there are many research trials (even medication trials) which use this as the measure—therefore it is a reasonable one to use.

It is important to note the dosing of the omega 3/6 supplements. Each subject took three capsules twice daily during the study, and active ingredients

---

4   *Journal of Attention Disorders* (2009) Johnson et al: "Omega-3/Omega 6 Fatty Acids for ADHD, A Randomized Placebo Controlled Trial in Children and Adolescents"; 12:5, p 394-401

were: EPA, 558 mg/day, and DHA, 174 mg/day. The brand name of the product studied was Eye Q.[5] If you decide to get Omega 3 supplementation from your local pharmacy or health food store, then just look for a supplement with a similar dose of active ingredients.

When it comes to Omega 3 supplementation, it is important to note that there are both plant sources and animal sources of Omega 3s. The plant sources are often derived from flax seed. While flax seed supplementation is being studied for how it helps with heart disease, arthritis and other medical conditions, it may be less effective for ADD and psychiatric issues. This relates to the fact that the plant-based Omega 3s have a shorter fatty acid chain. This chain is not long enough to travel across the blood-brain-barrier, and thus the plant-based Omega 3s don't help ADD. Short chain Omega 3s can be converted to long chain Omega 3s which can cross into the brain; however some research studies have shown that kids with ADD have less of that enzyme available, and thus they may be less efficient at doing that.

When Omega 3s come from fish sources, the Omega 3 fatty acid chains are long enough to cross into the brain. The main concern with getting a fish oil supplement is making sure that you get a pharmaceutical grade, mercury-free supplement.

When considering using Omega 3 supplementation, it is important to realize that it will take weeks or months to help, not days or weeks. Generally, there are very few side effects. Omega 3's can be taken on their own or at the same time as one takes medication. When considering the risk benefit ratio, there are very few risks, and potential benefits. The worst side effects may be: "fishy burps" (if the pill repeats on your child), the need to swallow a bigger gel capsule, and the costs of the supplement.

Omega 3s are also thought to decrease the clotting of platelets slightly. Platelets are the particles in our blood which start to make a clot before the scab is formed.

---

5   Eye Q is available at: www.equazen.co.uk.

If the platelets are less likely to clot, this will reduce the risk of heart disease and stroke—which is why Omega 3s are being researched in that clinical area as well. For the purposes of physically healthy kids and teens with ADD, a slight decrease in platelet clotting shouldn't have any impact on your child, unless there is some other medical issue or concern present. Talk to your doctor to be certain about the safety issue.

Regarding the dose of omega 3s to take, there are no clear instructions. Be aware that the total milligram dose on the bottle will reflect total fatty acids, and you want to be aware of the active ingredients. For example, a pill may have 1000 mg of fatty acids, yet the active EPA could only be 100 mg. Be sure to check the side of the bottle.

Omega 3 supplements often come as a large gel capsule. Many kids have trouble swallowing a pill that big. If you want to start omega 3s with a child who can't swallow, look for omega 3s in the following forms: liquid, chewable, or even "squirt" capsules. These will allow kids to take their supplements even if they can't swallow the bigger pills.

To find the different forms of omega 3 supplements, look in your local pharmacy, your local health food stores, or even local nutritional supplement stores (i.e. stores where guys who work out go to get protein powder). One of these locations should have a form of omega 3 supplement that will work.

Takeaways for Omega 3 Fatty Acid Supplementation

Omega 3s are showing early evidence for helping with ADD. There are few risks, and potential benefits. Remember:

* When getting Omega 3s, get a supplement which is fish based, not vegetable (i.e. flax).
* Ensure the supplement is pharmaceutical grade.
* Ensure the supplement is certified mercury free.

- The main active ingredients are EPA and DHA.
- One of the best studies done on omega 3s suggest taking the following dose per day: EPA 558 mg per day, DHA 174 mg per day.
- For children—look for liquid, chewable or "squirt" capsules.

Therapy #3: Homeopathy for ADD

Homeopathy is a therapeutic approach which often baffles western medical science. There appears to be no medical way that a homeopathic remedy can work. Homeopathy was developed by a German physician, Dr. Samuel Hahnemann in the late 18th century. He found that ingesting cinchona bark—which was used to treat malaria—actually caused him to experience certain symptoms which were similar to those of a patient suffering with malaria. He developed the "law of similars," which stated that remedies which caused symptoms would actually be helpful in treating them.

Dr. Hahnemann also found that if he diluted the substance substantially, its healing properties would remain, yet there would be few or no side effects. This is the law of "infinitesimality." To produce homeopathic remedies, the active ingredient is diluted in water, and then repeatedly diluted, while being shaken vigorously (which is referred to as *succussion*). When a homeopathic remedy is ready, scientists would not be able to find the original material left in the remedy, as it is diluted so much. In fact, in the homeopathic approach, the more dilute a substance is, the more powerful it is.

Although this makes no sense in the western medical model, practitioners of homeopathy refer to the fact that the memory or energy of the remedy is stored in the water/substance of the treatment. The analogy which is used is that of a CD ROM. If one were to analyze the CD ROM physically, one would find polycarbonite plastic and aluminum. And, based on physical analysis, a CD which contained the music of The Beatles would be the same as a CD which contained office software. However, the memory imprinted on the CD is different. This is how homeopaths view their remedies—that the water in the remedy has the imprint or memory of the remedy within it.

One of the other major principles of homeopathy is individualization. This refers to the fact that each individual requires different remedies and treatments, even if they have the same western medical diagnosis. This makes it very hard for research to be done on homeopathy, because of the fact that studies cannot be randomized.

When a homeopath is doing an assessment, he will go through your history in a lot of detail. You may be asked questions about things that seem unimportant, like whether your child gets cold hands and feet. All of these different symptoms help the homeopath to find the right remedy.

Once the history is taken, the homeopath refers to the "repertory," which is a reference which contains all of the different homeopathic remedies. The homeopath will find a remedy which seems helpful, and then find the right potency to help in the current situation.

Once this is all done, the homeopath recommends certain remedies, remedies which come as either a liquid, or small pills formulated with lactose.

Now that you have an overview of homeopathy, let's talk about the research for homeopathy in ADD. There was a Cochrane Collaboration Review of homeopathy in ADD in 2009.[6] The Cochrane Collaboration is a methodology to review the available science in a particular area to see if there is enough data to prove that a treatment is helpful. They use the scientific technique of meta-analysis.

In summary, the Cochrane Review of homeopathy found that there were no data to show that homeopathy works for ADD.

Why then do I still want to discuss homeopathy?

As mentioned above, homeopathy is a treatment which is not well suited to western medical clinical research. Even though the Cochrane Collaboration dismissed the results of homeopathic treatment, there is one study which really

---

caught my attention. One study is not enough to prove the effectiveness of any treatment, yet, for a treatment modality which is not well suited to clinical research, I felt that this was significant.

This study was completed in Switzerland. It was published in the journal *Homeopathy*[7] in 2007. This study could not be randomized initially. The experienced homeopathic physicians worked with children with ADD until they found a remedy which was helpful to them. This took on average five months, and there was a median of three different homeopathic medications tried to find a successful one. Once a remedy was found, the children were randomly switched to either placebo or the active treatment and followed going forward. After five months, there was a measurable difference between the group receiving placebo and the group receiving active homeopathic treatment.

To me, this study provided a possible direction of further research—some exciting understandings—about the potential for homeopathy in ADD. I don't dispute the scientific criticisms that the Cochrane Review make of this study. They are accurate. I just leave open the possibility that homeopathy is not well suited to current scientific methodology, and that there may be a treatment effect in ADD.

Takeaways regarding ADD and Homeopathy

Based on the research reviewed above, it is important to consult with a homeopathic physician who has a breadth of experience with homeopathy, and, hopefully, is experienced with ADD as well. Furthermore, it is important to realize that the results were measured after months of treatment, not days or weeks. If you are considering homeopathy, take these suggestions with you when developing your treatment plan.

---

7   *Homeopathy* (2007) Frei et al: "Randomized controlled trials of homeopathy in hyperactive children: treatment procedure leads to an unconventional study design."

Therapy #4: Herbal Treatments/Supplements

Many of the medicines which are used regularly today came from plant sources. For example, aspirin came originally from white willow bark. The cardiac medication, digitalis, came from the flower foxglove. Isn't it possible that herbal treatments can help with ADD?

If you are considering using herbal treatments or supplements for ADD, it is best to consult an expert. You may want to speak to an herbalist, a naturopathic doctor, or a Chinese medicine physician.

When looking into herbal treatments and supplements, there are no specific treatments for ADD as a medical diagnosis. One has to look at target symptoms, and then find a supplement to help with those. The most common target symptoms one aims to treat when working on ADD are: inattention/poor concentration, hyperactivity, impulsivity, and poor memory/short term memory problems.

There are very few studies with good data that indicate herbal treatments help ADD. There are some small studies which suggest there may be some help for ADD, though they are not conclusive.

Ginseng and Ginkgo Biloba for ADD

A combination of American Ginseng and Gingko Biloba was tested in a four week trial to see if it could help ADD.[8] The remedy used contained 200 mg of the American Ginseng extract *Panax quinquefolium*, as well as 50 mg of Gingko Biloba. The study had 36 children aged 3 to 17 who met the diagnosis of ADD. The herbal treatment was given twice daily on an empty stomach for four weeks. After four weeks, the researchers found that there was a 74 percent improvement on the main measure of ADD symptoms used in the study. While this sounds very impressive, because this was an open study, the results may not be reliable. In other

8   *Journal of Psychiatry Neuroscience* (2001) Lyon et al: "Effect of the herbal extract combination Panax quinquefolium and Ginkgo biloba on ADHD: a pilot study"; 26(3):221-8

words, there was no placebo arm to the study, and so we don't know if the effect of the treatment was really due to the treatment; it may be due to other factors (such as the parent's desire to see their child improve on an herbal treatment). This study, however, is still important because, though it is a preliminary study, it indicates that further research may be helpful.

Siberian Ginseng has data that it may help with enhancing concentration and memory in a three month study, a study that was done with adults and not in children. It is not clear that it is safe to use Siberian Ginseng in children or teens. This is where consulting with a professional would be helpful.

Pycnogenol for ADD

Pycnogenol is an extract of the maritime pine tree which grows exclusively along the coast of southwest France. It is an antioxidant and free radical scavenger. It is also thought to be a vasodilator (meaning that it opens up the blood vessels), which then allows the amount of blood flowing to the brain to increase, which can help with ADD symptoms.

There have been two randomized controlled trials of pycnogenol in ADD. There is one study with kids, and one with adults. In the child study, there was significant improvement in the teacher ratings of ADD symptoms, but in the adult study, there was no effect found. Interestingly, in the adult study, there were no effects, even in the group of the study which was taking methylphenidate medicine. This suggests that there was a study design problem, and that the results cannot be relied upon.

Some other possible remedies for ADD symptoms:

- There are some data that Gotu Kola can improve short term memory, as well as possibly anxiety.
- Valerian root is a natural "Valium." It helps to reduce anxiety, improve sleep and improve concentration.

There has been some research on using minerals for supplementation for ADD. These include: zinc, iron and magnesium.

Zinc for ADD

Zinc is a mineral which is needed for growth; this includes the immune system as well as neurological development. If your child is deficient in zinc, they can have cognitive impairments, and slow information processing.

A study in 2004 looked at using zinc as the only treatment for ADD.[9] It was a double blind, randomized, placebo controlled trial. The dose of zinc was 150 mg, and the study lasted for 12 weeks. The zinc group consisted of 202 children (107 of whom dropped out), and the placebo group consisted of 198 children (100 of whom dropped out). At the end of the study, zinc was found to be better for hyperactivity, impulsivity and impaired social issues—but it didn't help with inattention.

Another study looked at using zinc at 55 mg daily in addition to methylphenidate medication.[10] This study looked at 44 children aged five to 11 years old. It was a randomized, controlled trial. At the end of six weeks, it was found that the zinc led to better improvements than with a placebo when it was added to the methylphenidate medicine. This suggests that the zinc may boost the effects of the ADD medicine methylphenidate.

When it comes to considering using zinc as a supplement, it is important not to take too much. There are reports that at doses of 150 mg per day, there can be gastrointestinal side effects. And at doses of 300 mg daily, zinc can actually suppress the immune system. These side effects emphasize the importance of working with a professional when working with supplements, to ensure good response, and to minimize risks of side effects.

---

9   *Prog. Neuropsychopharmacol. Biol. Psychiatry* (2004) Bilici et al: "Double-blind, placebo controlled study of zinc sulfate in the treatment of ADHD"; 28(1), 181-190

10   *BMC Psychiatry* (2004) Akhondzadeh, S: "Zinc sulfate as an adjunct to methylphenidate for the treatment of ADHD in children: a double blind and randomized trial".

Iron for ADD

Iron has been considered as a treatment for ADD. It is known that if one is iron deficient (i.e. anemic), then there can be a decrease in attention. There were two studies —quite small—which showed there may be a benefit when taking iron supplementation for ADD. The main concern with iron: if you take too much iron supplementation, there can be serious cardiac side effects. Be sure to talk to your doctor and other health care professionals. It is my opinion that if there is no iron shortage (i.e. anemia), then the risks of taking iron for ADD likely outweigh the benefits.

Magnesium for ADD

Magnesium is another mineral which can be helpful in ADD. Magnesium plays a role in neurotransmitter synthesis (i.e. your brain cells creating the neurotransmitters which are needed to work properly). In 1997, Kozielec did a study which found a magnesium deficiency in 95 percent of 116 kids with ADD (aged nine to 12 years old). The magnesium deficiency was found by means of testing blood serum, red blood cells and hair with atomic absorption spectroscopy. Magnesium was supplemented in these kids over six months, and benefits were noted. Magnesium was found to improve the hyperactivity in ADD kids in the study. The dose of magnesium used was three mg per pound of weight per day (i.e. for a 50 lb child, the dose of magnesium was 150 mg/day). Again, remember to check with your health care professional before starting on any dose of a supplement.

Melatonin for Sleep

Melatonin is a supplement which can be taken to help with sleep. Our brains make melatonin, from our pineal gland. Melatonin is important in regulating day and night cycles.

Before humans had electricity, when the sun was up, the brain stopped making melatonin. When the sun went down, the brain would make melatonin, and it would make people sleepy. In our modern era, artificial light can be on all day and night, and thus our brains may not be able to create melatonin to regulate the day-night cycle properly (and I certainly see many teens in my office that spend all night up on their computers, video games or watching TV, and then sleep all day). When one takes a melatonin supplement, it may help your son or daughter to fall asleep. Generally, there are few if any side effects. Because melatonin is "natural," it is often easier to take than having to consider a pharmaceutical.

When it comes to dosing melatonin, I generally recommend starting at three mg, and progressing up to a maximum of nine mg. Take it about one hour before bedtime, and then adjust it as you see fit. While it generally comes in pills, there are other formulations, including liquid, melt-in-the-mouth pills, etc. Melatonin can be taken with stimulant medications—to improve the insomnia, which can be a side effect (of course the stimulant is taken in the morning, and the melatonin is taken at night). Be sure to talk with your doctor if you are going to take melatonin.

Takeaways for Herbal Treatments and Supplements for ADD

- Herbal treatments generally aim to help one of the symptoms of ADD: for example, inattention, hyperactivity, or memory problems.
- American Ginseng and Ginkgo Biloba may help ADD.
- Pycnogenol may help ADD symptoms in kids.
- Zinc supplementation can help with ADD symptoms on its own, or it may help methylphenidate medicine to work more effectively when it's taken in combination.
- Iron supplementation has little data that it helps—but be very careful about taking too much (i.e. it can be lethal).

- Magnesium supplementation was found to be helpful when it was given to kids with ADD who were found to be deficient in magnesium (which was 95 percent of the kids in the study).

- Melatonin can be taken to help with sleep.

Therapy #5: Neurofeedback for ADD

Researchers have been measuring brain waves of people with ADD for quite some time. To fully understand the impact of ADD on brain waves, let's review some basic information about brainwaves first.

When an EEG (electro-encephalogram) is attached to the scalp, it can measure the electrical brainwaves going through the brain. The frequency of the brainwaves provides an indication about someone's level of awareness or alertness. For example, there are four frequency ranges of brainwaves: alpha, beta, theta and delta. They are listed in Table 6 by their frequency range and associated mental state:

TYPE OF BRAINWAVE	FREQUENCY	MENTAL STATE
Beta	12-38 hz	Higher level concentration
Alpha	8-12 hz	Daydreaming
Theta	3-8 hz	Light sleep/meditation
Delta	0.2-3 hz	Deep sleep

Table 6: Brain waves: type, frequency range and associated mental state

As you can see in Table 6, as the brainwave frequency range is reduced, one goes from an alert state, through two intermediate stages, to a state of deep sleep.

Researchers who have looked at brainwaves in ADD have found that people with ADD spend more time in theta than other people do. In other words, when they should be focusing—i.e. in beta—they are actually in alpha (day dreaming) and in theta brainwaves.

Biofeedback is a process whereby people are trained to become aware of and ultimately able to manipulate unconscious processes. This can be done for heart rate and pain perception, as well as brain waves. The process of biofeedback for brainwaves is referred to as "neurofeedback."

To receive this treatment, you'll need to find a center which specializes in EEG neurofeedback. The process involves an initial assessment, and then the initiation of treatment. The treatment sessions consist of regular sessions (once or twice per week) for a total of up to 40 sessions. In each session, your child is connected to EEG wires (which are attached to electrodes adhering to their scalp) to measure their brainwaves. Just to be clear, these wires only sense the electrical activity of the brain; they don't actually transmit electricity to the brain. Then, your child is given some tasks to complete. When their brain waves are in beta (i.e. the active concentration brain state), then they receive positive reinforcement—for example, a car on a computer screen could move forward. As the reward / positive reinforcement occurs, it gradually trains your son's brain to spend more time in beta brainwaves rather than alpha or theta.

In January 2005, the Child and Adolescent Clinics of North American published an article reviewing the data on neurofeedback in ADD.[11] They reviewed four well designed studies, which showed promise for this treatment. They concluded that it would be impossible to conclude that neurofeedback is a proven treatment for ADD based on these studies; but they recommend larger, randomized trials to look for a true effect. The studies reviewed did show that about 75 percent of the participants did receive some benefit from neurofeedback. Additionally, the majority of individuals were able to reduce their ADD medications because of the neurofeedback treatment. They did not stop their medication, but adding neurofeedback gave them the ability to lower their dose.

---

11   *Child Adolesc Psychiatric Clin N Am 14* (2005) Gruzelier, J: "Critical validation studies of neurofeedback"; p.83– 104

In 2006, a fascinating study was completed about neurofeedback in ADD.[12] This study took 20 ADD children, and gave them 40, one-hour sessions of neurofeedback training. The kids were eight to 12 years old, and they were randomized to receive either neurofeedback or wait list control. One of the most unique features of this study was the fact that the researchers did fMRI studies before and after treatment. fMRI refers to "functional MRI." This is a strategy seeking to image the brain's activity while the child is performing a cognitive task. fMRI shows which parts of the brain are active. In this study, the kids were checked with fMRI before receiving treatment. After the neurofeedback treatment, the fMRI tests were repeated.

In this study, the neurofeedback provided significant improvement in the ADD symptoms compared to the wait list control. However, the most fascinating finding was the fact that the brain activity was much improved in the neurofeedback treated group based on their follow up fMRI tests. This suggests that not only does neurofeedback improve the symptoms of ADD, but it may also improve the efficiency of brain functioning of those with ADD.

The main criticism of this study relates to the fact that there was no active control—in other words the kids who did not receive neurofeedback, were just kept on a wait list. Therefore, it is possible that just sitting in front of a computer with a therapist without neurofeedback going on could lead to these benefits (this is unlikely, but a valid criticism of this study). A newer study was done to help to take this concern out of the equation.

In this newer study, published in 2009, the researchers compared active neurofeedback treatment to a different computer training program, with the desire to have a "control group."[13] In this study design, children were randomized

---

12   *Neuroscience Letters* (2006) Levesque, J et al: "Effect of neurofeedback training on the neural substrates of selective attention in children with AD/HD: A functional magnetic resonance imaging study"; 394, 216-221

13   *Journal of Child Psychology and Psychiatry* (2009). Gevensleben, et al.:" Is neurofeedback an efficacious treatment for ADHD? A randomized controlled clinical trial."

to receive either real neurofeedback, or they were receiving time on a computer training program where they were not receiving actual neurofeedback. This allows for a much better comparison between the active treatment (neurofeedback) and the other treatment—which was computer work—but it was not neurofeedback.

In this study, there were 102 children aged eight to 12 years old. About 80 percent were boys. They were all diagnosed with ADD, and over 90 percent had never taken medication for ADD.

At the end of the study, the group which received neurofeedback was significantly improved compared to the control group. They were improved based on parent-reported and teacher-reported ADD symptoms. The researchers also found that the neurofeedback group had lowered ratings of oppositional defiant disorder symptoms compared to the control group.

Because of its design, this study lends a lot of credibility to neurofeedback treatment for ADD. While there will still be people who criticize this study, and more research is needed, this study helps to pave the way for neurofeedback to receive the recognition it needs as a treatment for ADD.

Are there side effects for neurofeedback?

It is my contention that there are always side effects to effective treatments. In the case of neurofeedback, the only side effects that I can think of are time and money. In other words, you will have to invest time to go to the 40 sessions, and you will have to invest money to get the treatment done. No treatment is perfect, and even if there is a 75 percent chance of the treatment working, there is still a chance it won't work. My advice is to go into the treatment with your "eyes open" to these risks and then you can make an informed decision.

Takeaways for Neurofeedback

- Kids and teens with ADD often spend more time in theta brain waves, rather than beta (alert and focused) brain waves.

- Neurofeedback is a treatment which can improve kids with ADD's focus, as well as their brain activity (based on the fMRI study described above).
- A recent trial which was randomized and had a control group showed much more conclusive evidence that neurofeedback works for ADD.

Therapy #6: Cerebellar Treatments

There has been a newer approach to therapy for ADD which, however, is controversial. It is the cerebellar treatments.

The cerebellum is a small part of the brain at the back of the head. I learned in medical school that it is involved with motor (muscle) coordination. New brain research in ADD is showing that the cerebellum is actually involved in the symptoms of inattention, and not just motor/muscle coordination.

The cerebellar treatments were developed based on the recognition that there are differences in the cerebellum in people with ADD vs. people who don't have ADD. Mr. Wynford Dore was a British business man whose daughter was diagnosed with severed dyslexia. He began to research a drug-free treatment program for her. His research led him to develop the "Dore method," a system of physical exercises designed to improve the functioning and connections of the cerebellum. His contention was that these exercises improve symptoms of dyslexia, dyspraxia, learning disabilities, and ADD.

The treatment program is individualized, and it is not revealed to the public. It is treated as a commercial secret. It involves simple practical physical exercises. The exercises are personalized, based on testing. It is recommended that people do the exercises twice daily for 12 months.

Regarding the research on the Dore program—there has been significant controversy. There were some studies done showing improvement, though there has been significant criticism regarding the methodology used. The scientific and medical community felt that the conclusions (i.e. that the Dore method works) were not substantiated by the research done. Primarily, the conclusions that the Dore program treats ADD, dyslexia, Asperger's and more were not substantiated by the research.

For scientific papers, there is a summary of the treatment published by Bishop in 2007 where he shows the flaws of the research done to support the Dore program.[14] Reynolds published a follow up paper to support the exercise treatment.[15] In it, she documents ongoing improvement in people who have taken the treatment—with the benefits lasting as long as 18 months. This study documents improvements in cognitive (thinking) and motor (muscle) tasks. This study was done with a group of children who were "at risk" of dyslexia. They found benefits both in the children who were actually diagnosed with dyslexia and the children who were not diagnosed with dyslexia. There is no mention of ADD in this study.

There has also been controversy regarding the Dore center(s) themselves. The cost of treatment in the UK is £2000 (approximately $3000 US Dollars). The center has also gotten in trouble with the Advertising Standards Authority (ASA) in the UK for making unsubstantiated claims in their advertising. The ASA suggested that there were no data to support ads saying that the Dore method cured ADD, Dyslexia, Asperger's, etc. And the centers were closed in 2008 due to financial problems. They have since been bought, and re-opened.

Where does this leave you with respect to exercise training?

This is an unproven treatment at best. It may provide benefit to individuals who try it, though I'd love to see some controlled trials in defined populations before giving it a strong endorsement for ADD.

---

14   *J Paediatr Child Health*. 2007 Oct.: "Curing dyslexia and attention-deficit hyperactivity disorder by training motor co-ordination: miracle or myth?"; 43(10):653-5 Bishop, D.V.

15   *Dyslexia*. 2007 May, Reynolds: "Follow-up of an exercise-based treatment for children with reading difficulties"; 13(2):78-96.

In this circumstance, the biggest "side effects" to this treatment are time and money. You have to decide if it is worth investing your resources (time and money) into a treatment like this.

One last issue with the Dore centers—there are few of them around. Therefore, it is likely that you don't have access to a Dore center, even if you want to try it out. Furthermore, it is not the only cerebellar treatment available.

The Interactive Metronome®

The "Interactive Metronome®" is a software training program which is done at a therapy center. It involves training motor planning and sequencing. The patient does exercises which work on the timing of tapping and moving in time with rhythmic beats. The theory is that the brain is trained to do better with its planning and sequencing. When the planning and sequencing improves, this will help with thinking, planning and attention in real life.

There is a well designed study published in 2001 about the Interactive Metronome® in ADD.[16] It looked at 56 boys who were six to 12 years old with ADD. They were randomized to receive either the Interactive Metronome® treatment, training on another computer program, or just a control group with no active treatment. At the end of the study, there was a significant improvement for the boys who had ADD compared to the other groups. Their improvement was with attention, motor control, language processing, reading and the ability to regulate aggression. While this study is positive for the treatment, and well designed, it would be helpful to see more research done to replicate the findings and increase the confidence in this treatment. If you want to learn more about Interactive Metronome® treatment, visit their site at *www.InteractiveMetronome.com.*

---

16   *American J of Occupational Therapy* (2001) Shaffer et al: "Effect of Interactive Metronome Training on Children with ADHD."

The Learning Breakthrough Program

The Learning Breakthrough program is another program which is based on doing exercises to improve coordination, with the expectation that it will help learning and ADD. This program consists of a box of materials that is purchased, and all of the exercises are done at home. The current cost is $400 US dollars plus shipping. It is recommended that the exercises be done for 10 to 20 minutes twice daily for nine to 12 months.

The Learning Breakthrough program looks promising, and its website is very well designed, user friendly, and full of great multimedia to teach you about the program. It is very professional, and contains great endorsements—both from previous clients, and from well known thought leaders/doctors in the field. My main concern with the Learning Breakthrough Program is the lack of research documenting that their specific treatment actually works in ADD. Their website lists numerous studies which relate to the theoretical background of how it may work,[17] but there are no studies examining this treatment approach in ADD kids or teens.

Takeaways for Cerebellar Treatments

While there has been a lot of press and discussion about cerebellar treatments for ADD, there is a real shortage of research done to prove that it actually works. As such, it is hard to recommend this treatment modality. If you are interested, consider doing your own reading and reviewing of these programs to decide if it is worth it to invest your time and money in these programs. As I've mentioned in discussing previous alternative treatments—the biggest side effect for these programs is time and money. If you are able to decide that it may be worth it, you could choose to invest in these programs for the potential benefits. Just go

---

17   http://www.learningbreakthrough.com/topical-research-selections; accessed September 2010

in asking the right questions, and knowing that the treatment may not help your son or daughter.

Therapy #7: Software for Working Memory Training (Cogmed)

Cogmed is a new, software based, training program which is designed to improve working memory. Working memory refers to a specific executive function.

As we defined in Step 1 of the Attention Difference Disorder System, executive functions are the cognitive (thinking) processes that allow us to plan, prioritize and organize. They are the highest level of thinking. ADD is often thought to be a disorder of the executive functions.

Working memory refers to the ability to hold a small bit of information in your mind long enough to use it for problem solving. For example, if someone gives you a phone number, and you are holding that number in memory for several seconds as you are getting a pen—that is your working memory. If a student is listening to a teacher and writing down what she is saying—he is using his working memory. For example, if the teacher says "phrase one," the student begins to write down phrase one. While the student is still writing phrase one, the teacher is now saying phrase two. The student has to hold in working memory what the teacher has said in phrase two while finishing writing phrase one, etc.

Some people theorize that working memory problems are in fact the biggest deficit in ADD, and if we can fix them, then we will improve functioning in ADD overall.

Cogmed is a software training program which is designed to train working memory. There are specific memory tasks which are performed on a home computer five days per week over a period of five weeks. Each homework session is approximately 30 minutes long. The difficulty level of the software exercises is determined by the individual's initial assessment, and then it is increased according to an algorithm.

To take part in Cogmed, you need to find a Cogmed center close to you. The cost is in the $1500 range, and you will visit with the Cogmed professional to get started. You will have weekly contact with the therapist as you progress through the treatment.

Cogmed has had impressive research completed and published about its program. One of the best studies for Cogmed and ADD was published in 2005 in the *Journal of the American Academy of Child and Adolescent Psychiatry*.[18] In this study, 53 ADD children were studied, who were not on medication, 44 completed the training, and 42 of them were evaluated three months later. The kids were randomly assigned to either active treatment, or a comparison software program which did not provide treatment. The main outcome measure was improvement on a working memory test (which was not part of the training—to avoid a "learning effect").

This study showed that Cogmed had a significant treatment effect both right after the treatment was finished, as well as at follow-up at three months. The working memory was improved, and there were findings that other measures had also improved, including: verbal working memory, response inhibition, complex reasoning and parent-rated inattention.

This and other studies show that Cogmed is a potential treatment option for ADD. Does it work for all kids and teens with ADD?

I'm not sure that we know the answer to that. My impression is this: if your son or daughter has significant executive functioning difficulties (i.e. problems with working memory, planning, organization, prioritizing, etc.) then it is likely that Cogmed may help. It is also important to note that even if your child is taking medication, it is possible that the Cogmed program may help in a different way than the medication does. Research has shown that sometimes executive functions are not improved with medication, and if this is the case, Cogmed may help with treatment for these symptoms.

---

18   *J Am Acad Child Adolesc Psychiatry* (2005) Klingberg, T: "Computerized training of working memory in children with ADHD - A randomized controlled trial."

What are the drawbacks of Cogmed?

As previously mentioned with other alternative treatments, there are the possible side effects of time and money. In addition to that, for the treatment to work, you have to get your child to complete the software training on a daily basis for 30 to 40 minutes, five days per week. For some families, this can be a challenge. If you are interested but concerned about this issue, contact your local Cogmed provider and ask for suggestions on how to handle this. (Your local Cogmed provider can be found by visiting *www.cogmed.com* and clicking on "find a practice.")

Takeaways for Cogmed

Cogmed is a software-based working memory training program which can improve executive functioning, as well as symptoms of ADD. You will need to get your child to do 30 to 40 minutes of software training five days per week for five weeks. There is good research to support the use of Cogmed in ADD. You can find out more, and find a local provider at: *www.cogmed.com*

Summary Points for Step 6: Alternatives for ADD

In this section, we have covered many different options for alternative approaches to treatment with ADD. Each has different amounts of research to back up its use, and ultimately, you, your family, your child or teen and your healthcare practitioners will have to decide what is right for your situation and treatment. Here are some summary points to remember with respect to alternatives:

1. When considering alternative treatments for ADD, consider taking an approach of complementary treatment rather than alternative treatment. In other words, consider adding these treatments to standard medical care, rather than using them as an alternative—which would involve disregarding standard medical treatment.

2. Please have good discussions with your doctor about it. Most people do not communicate with their doctor about alternatives, and it's my belief that it hinders their treatment. Use this chapter as a resource if needed, and you may need to educate your doctor. It's worth it. And, if your doctor is closed-minded and dismisses the proposition, you can decide how to handle that later on. Hopefully you can find a more open-minded doctor.

3. Get the best research on the alternative treatments that you can. You've started here, and now you should do research in many other locations as well.

4. Whenever you are trying any treatment, make sure to have active monitoring of the effectiveness of the treatment. Whether it is medicine or diet change, you need to monitor if it is working, and adjust it as needed. Ideally your medical practitioner can help you to monitor the treatment response over time.

5. View ADD treatment as a marathon, not a sprint. Make sure to "pace yourself" and make decisions with the perspective of the fact that you will be dealing with ADD for months and years, not days or weeks, Remember to keep track of any risks or impairment which can be interfering with your child's functioning.

6. Even if you aren't sure where to start with alternatives, or whether they are for you, I suggest you start adding Omega 3 fatty acid supplements to your child's daily routine. They are quite low risk for side effects and have a good potential upside. Refer to the Omega 3 section above to review the dosing recommendations.

7. Start making simple diet changes. As described above in the diet change section, even if you aren't sure about doing a complete elimination diet,

work towards cutting out simple carbohydrates and food additives. Even if there isn't strong data for this in the research, it is healthy nutrition which means healthy living, and there is no harm from that. And it may just help the ADD as well.

8. Get regular exercise. New research is being done which shows that exercise is very good for the brain—even for ADD. Ensure that your child gets regular exercise. It creates better blood flow to the brain, and can help with sleep and stress. If your child is stuck on the couch playing video games, see if you can enroll him in an activity that he'll enjoy: karate, sports teams, or even solo exercise like running. And if he's reluctant, see if you can keep physical education as a credit on his school schedule.

9. Finally, I encourage you to seek out local resources to learn more about alternative treatments in your area. Parent support groups may have the information that you need to make decisions about treatments which will help your child. Do the research; make the local connections; and see if you can find a professional to help you to navigate the different alternative treatment options which may help you with your ADD son or daughter.

CHAPTER 9

Step 7: Treatment Integration

a t this point, we have covered the major steps in the Attention Difference Disorder System which help you to turn your ADD child or teen's differences into strengths in seven steps. We have covered:

1) Step 1: Education about ADD

2) Step 2: Ensuring a proper assessment

3) Step 3: Parenting Strategies for ADD

4) Step 4: School and Academic Strategies

5) Step 5: Medication Treatment for ADD

6) Step 6: Alternative Treatments for ADD

The final step is about bringing it all together. Treatment integration is all about integrating the different treatments at different times as needed.

When ADD is first diagnosed, it can be quite overwhelming for parents to make sense of it all. There is a lack of knowledge, a sense of guilt (i.e. did I cause this; is it my fault?), worry about making the right choices (should I give medication, or should I not give medication?), and the need to interact with other adults or professionals about your child—the staff at his school, for example.

And once the ADD seems settled and on track, your child goes and grows up another year or two, and the things that worked before don't seem to be working anymore. Parents often will say to me: "Is his behavior worse because something's wrong, or is it just the testosterone from puberty?" You need to be constantly adjusting the treatment to suit your child's growth and development.

If ADD treatment were a recipe, once you get the recipe right, it is only a short time before it doesn't seem to be working out, and you are "back to the kitchen,"

There are several factors which impact the treatment of ADD over time. These include:

1. The decisions you make, and the approaches you take
2. The resources available in your community
3. Growth and development over time
4. Social and family factors
5. School factors
6. The co-existing conditions which may be present now, or which may come in the future.

Treatment integration is a very important part of succeeding with ADD over time. It is often left out in other books and resources for parents.

Factor 1: The Decisions You Make and the Approaches You Take

As your child is diagnosed, and you are getting recommendations from your health care practitioners, you will begin to make decisions about the approach that you want to take.

Even if you completely agree with everything written about in the Attention Difference Disorder seven step system, from a practical perspective you will need to choose what to implement first and what can wait. For some families, starting with parenting approaches is critical. For other families, it may be school strategies as well as medication as the first step. And yet other families may begin with alternative treatments and getting more education about ADD and its impact.

This is where it is particularly important for you to have treatment discussions with a healthcare team that you trust. I know from experience that there are many people who do not have a doctor with enough expertise in ADD. There either isn't one in their community, or it isn't covered by their insurance, or the doctor isn't taking any new referrals.

As you take advice from your healthcare professionals, think about your current treatment decisions, and also think two steps ahead. If you are starting with parenting and medication, get all of the information you need about these treatments, and get educated about what can happen after that. Ask your doctor about monitoring the medicine over time. Consider what can happen with school strategies once you get things more under control at home. Consider where alternative approaches can fit in once the timing is right.

As with any complex task—it takes planning. And treating ADD is a complex task. ADD can be a challenging disorder, and it can change so much over time.

One of the goals of this book is to give you a complete overview of the treatment needed. Once you are educated enough to make informed choices about which approaches to take, you can then decide which order to implement them in.

Your course of treatment for ADD may be different than your friend's course of treatment for ADD. That course will be based on the treatments you start with and how they work. Keep this in mind—and realize that the treatment of ADD can be a moving target over time.

Factor 2: The Resources Available in Your Community

There is often a significant shortage of services for ADD (and mental health in general) in many communities. Mental health is often treated like the "black sheep" of the medical family, particularly when it comes to funding and fundraising. The fact that there is still stigma and ignorance out there about ADD and mental health in general perpetuates this problem.

As the parent of a child or teen with ADD, you have to search for the best resources which are available to you in your community. You may start with the doctor, and then include other resources like a psychologist, occupational therapist (if needed), speech and language therapist (if needed), social worker, family therapist, school staff, tutors/special education teachers, alternative health care providers, and more.

You'll need to start with the resources you can get easily, and do your best. As time goes on, keep your "ear to the ground" for new resources—i.e. maybe a new ADD clinic is opened in your community or a Cogmed provider opens up, etc. Keeping in touch with the local parents and support groups can help tremendously in this regard.

The reality for most families is that you will have to work with what you've got. Most families won't be able to choose a different school, or a private school. You will have to go into your child's school and get the best resources that you can. And this may mean becoming a great advocate, and educating the professionals in the school as to how to handle ADD. Remember your "Parent's ADD Journey":

Student➔ Expert➔ Advocate

It shouldn't have to be this way, but it may just be, nevertheless. I encourage you to take a proactive, non-judgemental approach—i.e. focus on *the outcome* of your child getting the help that she needs, rather than the process of how many meetings will be needed to get your child the help that is necessary.

Remember that it may be possible to get some help from other areas. A treatment like coaching can make a difference for teens with ADD, and it can be delivered over the telephone. This way, you can get the benefit of help without close physical proximity. Also—if you don't have a local parent support group, you can find one online, and benefit from the expertise of parents from other parts of your state, country, or even internationally.

Factor 3: Growth and Development over Time

This is a critically important factor. The issues which a child faces with ADD are different at just about every developmental stage. The issues at six years old are different than they are at eight, and 10, and even at 16 years of age. You need to be prepared for the fact that things will change, and you will have to adapt the treatment approach for ADD.

In early childhood, the major tasks for your child are to get into a successful learning approach with school, to start to handle routines and behaviors at home, and to develop socially. Different kids have different challenges with each of these areas, and you'll need to adjust treatment to support your child. One of the big issues that happens around six to eight years old is that the social interactions become more complicated and complex. This can lead to your son having trouble relating to friends. When kids are in kindergarten, it's OK to just "zoom cars" next to each other, but as kids grow, their social interactions become more complex. Be sure to keep on the lookout for social issues.

As kids begin to go through puberty, they now have a lot of hormones impacting their thinking and behavior. This is put on top of the increasing challenges of school, other activities, and the increasing complexity of social interactions (they start to become aware of their sexuality and they become interested in potential sexual partners).

Adolescence can be hard enough to handle without ADD, and you need to be prepared to work to adapt treatment and support your child during their adolescence. Remember to constantly make deposits into the "bank of connection" between you and your child (as we covered in Step 3, "Parenting Strategies for

ADD"). It is the connection that your child feels to you which can help him to trust your support during the potentially difficult teen years.

Entering high school is one of the biggest transitions and changes that a teen will make. And it can lead to real challenges. You see, when teens get to high school, they enter a truly unstructured time in their education. There is no one to look over their shoulder and make sure that they've done all that they are supposed to do. If they have organizational problems, this can lead to a lot more trouble. If you are able to put the necessary supports in place before high school, this can make a big difference.

And of course, your job as a parent doesn't end when your child is 18 years old. If your teen still has ADD as he's entering adult life, there are a whole new set of challenges. These challenges are very important, yet they are beyond the scope of this book.

In summary, as your child grows and develops, there will be changes to the treatment needed—and you will need to be flexible and on top of the monitoring of your child's progress and symptoms to react quickly and proactively.

Factor 4: Social and Family Factors

Social factors refer to the social issues which affect your family. These can relate to your family's living situation, income, the people who live with you, as well as the insurance coverage you have for your medications, or therapies.

Over the course of your child or teens life, there can be many changes. Separations and divorces can happen. Other siblings can be born, or can be diagnosed with ADD. Illnesses, job losses, and other challenges can arise. This is life—and it happens to all of us.

As different challenges arise in your family, you'll need to remember that your child with ADD may need extra help or support to handle the changes. He may not be as flexible as needed, and it may take longer for him to adjust to the new situation.

Tightly intertwined with social factors are different family factors. This can refer to changes in relationships—i.e. when a single mom remarries—an ADD child can take longer to adjust to the new family unit. Or it can relate to challenges with the extended family. I often hear about challenges in divorced families with joint custody—where the Mom gives medicine on weekdays, and works hard on the treatment, and then Dad refuses to give medicine and undermines the treatment. Family support can be incredibly helpful, and also, unfortunately, family challenges can be particularly undermining.

Consult your healthcare team about the best way to support your child if a major social change affects the family, and if you are having particular family challenges.

Factor 5: School Factors

Getting the right support at school is very important, and it can also be challenging, as we covered in Chapter 6, Step 4, "School and Academic Strategies for ADD."

There are many parents who work hard with the school to get the right supports into place, and then changes can happen. The changes may be a result of your child moving to a new school, or it could be that the staff at the school changes, and this can impact the support that your son or daughter gets.

If you do have to move schools, there are many parents who find this a challenge, because of the fact that they feel that they have to start all over again with the new school—i.e. to ensure that their child is getting the support he or she needs. However, remember that there are times that a new school may provide better support and help to your child or teen.

There can also be staffing changes which can impact your child or teen's supports in school. The principal who was so helpful could be moved to another school, or the special education teacher retires. When these things happen, it can be hard, because you may feel that the replacement isn't providing the same level of support or understanding for your child, and you feel that it has set you back. While this may be the case, remember that "life happens" and one of the long-term treatment goals for your child is to develop the ability to adapt and to be flexible. Just do your best to get the new staff to understand your child and his or her needs.

Of course, as any student goes through school, there are changes which happen naturally. For example, all students are expected to work more independently as they progress through their education. There are some ADD students who do reasonably well until they get farther in school— i.e. they may struggle with the "transitional years," meaning the years they go from elementary school to middle school, or from middle school to high school. During these years, the expectations on them are greater, and it may overwhelm their ability to cope. During these times, you may need to ensure that there is extra support and treatment in place to make sure that they don't lose the progress that they've made and start to do poorly.

Also remember that in high school, all teens are exposed to more risky situations. First of all, there is less direct monitoring of them, so they feel that they can get away with more, and may get into bad habits like skipping school.

High school is also a time when students can get involved with more risky behaviors—such as drinking alcohol, using cigarettes, marijuana or other street drugs, and getting involved in sex. If an ADD teen feels frustrated and angry a lot of the time—who do you think that he or she is going to spend time with? The students who go to the library and do all of their school work, or the students who hang around in the "smoking pit," skip school, and get into risky behavior? This is one of the reasons that you want to help your child as early as possible, so that he or she is more likely to be on track both academically and socially. This is also why you need to build on the "bank of connection" we spoke about in Chapter 5, Step 3, "Parenting for ADD." If you can maintain good communication with your ADD teen, you may be able to be a resource to him when he has questions or concerns about these risky situations (around drugs, sex, driving, etc.). Realize that a teen has to feel quite comfortable to bring these issues up with his parent, and that is why you need to work hard to have effective parenting strategies, and you need to build your relationship with your child.

During high school, your child will also need to put some serious thought into what he or she may want to do in the future. While this can be quite anxiety inducing for teens, it is an important area which needs to be addressed. It is important for your teen to explore different areas of interest, and it is very important for parents of an ADD teen to do their best to provide opportunities for their ADD teen to get some experience in areas of their interest.

Maybe he is interested in photography, and a family friend is a photographer, and would be willing to have him volunteer for two Saturdays to see what it is like to work as a real photographer. Or maybe he can work toward an apprenticeship in an area he loves, or have coffee with a family friend who is a lawyer to see if that is right for him. While this is important for all teens, it is even more important for teens with ADD.

If your teen is heading toward college or university, know that often times these post-secondary schools have better supports in place for students with ADD or other learning challenges. You can research the supports available at the different schools that your son or daughter is considering and ensure that the support is in place when your teen goes on to this stage of education. Your teen may also need more help in navigating the complicated applications process than other teens do.

One other major issue which comes up during adolescence and high school is driving. Many teens get their driver's licence, and this can be quite risky. One of the leading causes of death for older teens / young adults is motor vehicle accidents. It is very important that you monitor your teen's safety behind the wheel. I encourage you to have a "zero tolerance" policy for drinking or drug use around driving (which is the law anyway). It is also important to have a zero tolerance rule for not talking on the cell phone, not texting and not browsing the internet on their cell phones while driving (this is the law in many states as well). The early reports on the number of accidents caused by teens who are using their phones while driving is quite concerning.

I also encourage you to look at medication use while driving. If teens *without* ADD are at a high risk of motor vehicle accidents, then it is logical that teens *with* ADD are at an even higher risk—i.e. they are inattentive and impulsive behind the wheel of the car. This is an active area of research, and it is becoming clear that teens and young adults with ADD who are driving, are at a higher risk of citations and accidents. There is also research showing that with effective medication for ADD, these risks drop. Since many of the ADD medications wear off by early evening, talk to your doctor about a strategy for medication so that when your teen is returning home from a party after 11 pm, he will have medication in his system to help keep him safe behind the wheel. Though this strategy may not work for all families, I have had some families in my office who tell their teen that they can't use the car if they don't take their ADD medication—because it is too much of a safety issue.

Factor 6: Co-existing Conditions Which may Be Present Now, or Which may Come in the Future

This final factor is a very important one, and merits more time than the others. It starts with this simple rule of thumb with ADD: *ADD rarely comes alone.* This refers to the fact that up to 75 percent of kids and teens have at least one other diagnosis in addition to their ADD. And a high percentage of those kids have three or four diagnoses in addition to their ADD.

The proper medical term for an additional diagnosis is: a *comorbid* condition, and the overall term is *comorbidity*. This refers to the fact that the additional condition can lead to more "morbidity," or problems/challenges. As I feel that families with ADD often have to deal with enough negativity, I generally refer to these as "co-existing conditions."

Below are listed the approximate rates of co-existing conditions in ADD kids and teens. These rates are based on my reading of many different research papers.

COEXISTING CONDITION	APPROXIMATE RATE:
Oppositional Defiant Disorder	Up to 60 percent
Learning Disabilities	Up to 40 percent
Depression	Up to 35 percent
Anxiety Disorders	Up to 45 percent
Conduct Disorder	Up to 25 percent
Substance Abuse/dependence	Up to 30 percent

Table 7: ADD and the rates of co-existing conditions in kids and teens

As you review Table 7, you need to remember that it is possible for someone to have two or more disorders. That is why the rates do not add up to 100 percent—they go much higher than that. Allow me to be clear—I am not suggesting that your child will develop any or all of these conditions. However, to be thorough about ADD treatment, it is critical that you understand that there is a chance for a second or even third condition being present in your child. The importance for treatment integration is that the co-existing conditions have a big impact on how ADD treatment works. If treatment for simple ADD isn't working well, then it's possible there is a co-existing condition which hasn't been identified yet.

Specialists in ADD know that ADD becomes all about the co-existing conditions. In other words, how the treatment progresses often has a lot more to do with which co-existing conditions are present than the primary condition itself. For example, the symptoms and management are very different when there is ADD and Oppositional Defiant Disorder (ODD), vs. ADD and an anxiety disorder. This is also one of the biggest reasons why it is important for you to get a thorough assessment for ADD: to establish whether there are any co-existing conditions, or whether your child is at risk of any co-existing conditions developing shortly.

It's important to review the impact of the co-existing conditions on ADD. Feel free to read this whole section, or just read the section(s) which are relevant to you.

ADD and Behavior Disorders: The Implications for Treatment

There are two main behavior disorders which can come along with ADD. They are: oppositional defiant disorder (ODD) and conduct disorder (CD). ODD occurs in up to 60 percent of boys with ADD (it is lower with girls—in the 35 percent range), and conduct disorder occurs in up to 25 percent of kids with ADD.

ODD is a diagnosis which refers to kids who challenge authority. They are defiant. Conceptually, they go up to "the line" (that the adult is enforcing) and they step on the line, or torment the person holding the line. They don't actually cross the line. ODD's severity has a big impact on how it comes out in your child's life. If it is mild ODD, then your child is a bit more of a challenge, and can be more defiant than you like. If it is severe ODD, then it can rip your family apart—with anger, frustration and daily battles. ODD can impact your child in all realms—home, school and socially. There are times that parents are very upset that ODD only manifests at home. When this happens, I encourage parents to be grateful that their child's symptoms aren't spilling into the rest of his life, and work hard on what is going on at home.

When it comes to the treatment of ADD and ODD, the parenting strategies become critically important. The approach to discipline needs to be clear and implemented appropriately and regularly. If the ODD is manifesting at school, then the school has to be involved in the behavioral treatment as well.

Medication for ADD can help the ODD symptoms as well. For each of the major medicines, there have been research studies showing that when the ADD symptoms respond to the ADD medication, the ODD symptoms improve as well. There are times that doctors will consider using an add-on medication to help with significant ODD. Medicines like Intuniv˙, and other medicines in that group, like clonidine and guanfacine, can be helpful to settle behavior. Additionally, the medication risperidone can be helpful. Risperidone will be covered in the CD section.

Conduct disorder (CD) is a serious condition with significant public health implications. It refers to kids or teens who repeatedly break rules—including the rules of society. They engage in aggression (starting fights, bullying), theft, fire setting, hurting animals, breaking and entering, etc. This is, essentially, childhood criminal behavior. To meet the diagnosis of conduct disorder, a youth has to have at least three of the conduct disorder behaviors in the recent past. This means that if a teen is only caught shoplifting (which could just be an isolated impulsive act), then he does not necessarily have the diagnosis of CD.

When a child or teen meets the diagnosis of conduct disorder, there is a serious long term risk. Risks can be as high as 50 percent for later adult criminal behavior. If CD is present, then treatment needs to be more aggressive and deliberate. There are relatively few treatments which have been proven to work with CD. These include: a) treating coexisting conditions aggressively, b) multi-systemic therapy, and c) the medication risperidone.

When there is ADD and CD, it is really important to control the ADD as best as possible. The ADD could drive some of the impulsivity which causes the CD. If the ADD is well treated, it may lead to improvement. This is a situation where it would be better not to wait too long to use medication to treat the ADD. You'd want to treat the ADD, and increase the dose quickly to try to control the dangerous acting out behavior. If there are any other coexisting conditions as well—i.e. depression or anxiety, it is best to treat these as well. Talk to your doctor about the best approach.

The second proven treatment for CD is a program called multi-systemic therapy (MST). This is a well researched treatment which helps teens to not commit crimes, and to improve in other ways as well. It is proven to help, though it is only available in a relatively small number of locations. Talk to your doctor about whether it is available in your community, and if not, see if there is a therapist who has experience with conduct disordered kids who can use the principles of MST to help you out. You can read more about this treatment at the following website: *www.MSTServices.com.*

The third proven treatment to help CD is the medication risperidone. Risperidone is an "atypical antipsychotic." This is a newer generation antipsychotic medication. It was originally developed for schizophrenia and then it was also found to help with bipolar disorder, and the treatment of refractory depression. In child and adolescent psychiatry, risperidone has been proven to be helpful in autistic kids (particularly if they are aggressive) and conduct disordered kids. Please note: using risperidone in under 18 year olds is generally considered to be "off-label" usage. This means that this medication is not officially approved to be used in this age range for this condition. That said, most doctors will use it when it's needed because of the severity of and consequences from a conduct disorder.

Risperidone can be dosed once or twice daily. The doses generally start low (i.e. 0.25 mg or 0.5 mg). It is important to generally keep the dose below two mg daily. On occasion, a doctor may raise the dose above this level, but this is a general rule of thumb when risperidone is used in kids and teens. The most common side effects are fatigue and increased appetite, and upwards of 35 percent of kids/teens can gain weight when they take this medicine.

There are some rare but serious side effects with risperidone, like increasing the hormone prolactin (which can lead to lactation in boys or girls, and can stop girls' menstrual cycles). There have also been case reports of the medicine increasing cholesterol and triglycerides (which can be a long-term cardiovascular risk), as well as increasing blood sugar (which can either predispose someone to diabetes, or there have been case reports of it actually causing diabetes). Based on the side effects listed, the decision to take risperidone is an important one, and your doctor should monitor your child more closely if risperidone is used.

ADD and Learning Disabilities: Implications for Treatment

The first challenge when it comes to the combined learning disabilities (LD) and ADD, is that often they present a challenge to a complete diagnosis. Sometimes, doctors may diagnose one of these conditions, and then miss the other one. Sometimes parents feel that if their child is diagnosed with learning disabilities, then he doesn't have ADD as well—it is just part of the LD.

One of the other big challenges with ADD and LD's is how they are diagnosed. ADD can be diagnosed by a medical doctor—which is often covered by people's health insurance. Learning disabilities are diagnosed after complete psychoeducational assessments are made. These must be completed by psychologists, and may not be covered under people's insurance. They are quite costly. The school can provide this testing, though sometimes they do not have enough resources to test everyone, or the waiting list is too long. As we discussed in Step 4: School strategies for ADD, ideally each child with ADD would have a psychoeducational assessment. This would help to rule out any learning disabilities, and help to recognize your child's learning strengths and weaknesses, which can help with educational planning.

The bottom line if your child has both ADD and LD: you need to treat both in order to get the benefit from the treatment for either. If your child gets treatment for the LD (i.e. learning strategies and supports), but your child can't focus because of the untreated ADD, they won't benefit from the LD treatment. If they have treatment for ADD (i.e. strategies and/or medicine) so they can focus better, but they aren't getting help for the LD, then they can focus, but they are not benefiting from the teaching approach that is being given to them.

> **When ADD and LD are present together, make sure to pursue treatment for both.**

ADD and Depression: Implications for Treatment

ADD and depression can occur relatively frequently. Many people wonder if depression can actually be a consequence for untreated ADD—meaning that as a youth goes through life struggling (due to untreated ADD), it starts to affect their self esteem, which can ultimately lead to depression. While there is no clear research to prove this, it does make logical sense as a theory.

There are two main kinds of depression: major depressive disorder (major depression) and dysthymia. Major depression refers to the situation where there is a clear depressive episode that lasts for one week or longer, and involves excessive sadness, lack of interest or pleasure in activities, changes to sleep, appetite & concentration, loss of hope for the future, and may even include suicidal ideas or actions.

While a major depressive episode has to last for at least a week, it could last for a lot longer. It is important to note that when kids or teens have depression, they don't always have a depressed mood—they may have significant irritability instead of a depressed mood. Whereas depression is a major disruption over a short time, dysthymia is more of a low grade, sad mood that lasts for a lot longer. In kids and teens, it has to last for at least one year.

(Please note: the description of the diagnosis of depression is vague, sufficiently so, that you should make sure to talk to your doctor if you are worried about depression in your child or teen).

The biggest worry around depression is the risk of suicide. When depression is combined with ADD, you are now combining depressed mood, suicidal thoughts, and, potentially, impulsivity from the ADD. This can be a very concerning and disconcerting combination of symptoms (i.e. the risk is that he'll make an impulsive suicide attempt). If you are concerned about suicide risk, speak to your doctor or use your local emergency medical services to ensure your child's safety.

Treatment of depression involves a combination of medication and therapy. There are several different therapies which can help child and adolescent depression. At the top of the list is cognitive behavioral therapy (CBT). When it comes to medication, the first line medications used are generally the selective serotonin reuptake inhibitors (SRRI's), in particular prozac (fluoxetine). You need to be careful about using antidepressants in kids and teens because of the risk of causing suicidal ideas when these medicines are started (approximately a two percent risk). That said, the medicines can be quite safe and helpful—you just need to work with your doctor to ensure that there are appropriate safety measures and monitoring in place to help ensure the safety of your child.

Now that we've reviewed the treatment of depression, let's talk about what to do when it is present with ADD. If someone is just coming in for assessment, and they are diagnosed with ADD and depression, the doctor has to make a decision about which treatment should be started first—should we treat depression first, or ADD first. While there are no hard and fast rules, and the situation will be evaluated by your doctor (hopefully with your input), here are some general guidelines:

The doctor will usually pick the condition which either needs treatment first (because it is more severe), or the condition which will have the biggest impact on your child's functioning. For example, if there is a serious depression, with suicidal thoughts, then the doctor will treat the depression first, and deal with the ADD later (when the depression is more stable). If there is a more minor depression, which seems to come from the ADD symptoms (i.e. his sadness builds every time he does poorly on a test at school because he knows he can do better), then treating the ADD may help the ADD and the depression as well. Although this is a rough guideline, it will ultimately require a judgment call that the doctor and you will have to make together.

ADD and Anxiety: Implications for treatment

Anxiety disorders can be common in kids and teens with ADD. The anxiety disorders which can occur in kids include:

- **Generalized Anxiety Disorder (GAD):** This refers to excessive worrying, which is hard to control and interferes with functioning.

- **Social Anxiety Disorder:** This refers to serious shyness and an avoidance or severe difficulty with presentations, which interferes with functioning; it can also lead to school refusal.

- **Separation Anxiety Disorder:** This refers to serious anxiety when separating from a major caregiver.

- **Panic Disorder:** This refers to kids who get panic attacks which may not have a clear trigger.

- **Posttraumatic Stress Disorder (PTSD):** this refers to kids who have gone through a traumatic experience, and they have psychological consequences from that experience (nightmares, flashbacks, hypervigilance, fears, etc).

- **Specific phobias**: this refers to specific fears like spiders, lightening, heights, etc.

- **Obsessive Compulsive Disorder (OCD):** This refers to kids who have significant obsessions (recurrent intrusive thoughts) and compulsions (recurrent actions taken with the intention of relieving the obsession). Common actions include hand washing for germ obsessions, counting, perfectionism, etc.

Depending on your doctor's approach, she could diagnose two or three anxiety disorders (like GAD and Separation Anxiety Disorder together), or she may just say that your child has an "anxiety disorder" and leave it with just one diagnosis, meant to encompass all of the different symptoms.

The treatment for anxiety disorders is also a combination of medication and therapy. Similar to depression, the therapy which is proven to help with anxiety disorders is cognitive behavioral therapy (CBT), and the medications which can help are the SSRI's. The risk of causing suicidal ideas is still present when SSRI's are prescribed for anxiety disorders, and this should be reviewed and discussed with your doctor.

When ADD and anxiety are present together, the doctor will need to decide which disorder needs attention first. The doctor will pick the condition which either needs treatment first (because it is more severe), or the condition which will have the biggest impact on your child's functioning. For example, if there is severe anxiety which is preventing your child from going to school, or out of the house socially, then that will require immediate attention, and the ADD can be addressed later. If there is some anxiety on a day-to-day basis because your teen is forgetful, and she worries that things will go wrong because of it, then treating the ADD will actually have a positive effect on improving the anxiety.

One comment about medication in ADD and anxiety—while the stimulant medicines can be taken at the same time as the SSRI's for anxiety, there is good research that the non-stimulant Strattera˚ can treat both at the same time. (Please note: this applies to all of the anxiety disorders except OCD, which is harder to treat and doesn't seem to respond to Strattera˚.)

ADD and Substance Abuse or Dependence: Treatment Implications

Many teens in western countries experiment with drugs and alcohol during their adolescence. While this may be an overall concern, it becomes a lot more concerning when the "experimentation" with drugs or alcohol crosses over into a pattern which is concerning and interferes with a teen's life.

The difference between substance abuse and dependence: when a teen is abusing drugs or alcohol, it means that they are using it at a level which is more than they should. You could argue that anything beyond zero is more than they should (and you are right), though it is a fine line to establish whether the abuse is too much and leads to problems.

For example, if your teen ends up in the emergency room with alcohol poisoning—that is clearly too much. If your teen can't go to a party on the weekend and have fun unless they are drunk or high, that is too much. If your teen is not fulfilling major responsibilities because of the substance use—i.e. not attending school, or work—then that is too much. If your teen has two beers every few weekends with friends, that is likely not too much or problematic.

Substance dependence includes all of the aspects described above for substance abuse—plus it introduces tolerance, and withdrawal. Tolerance refers to the fact that the same response is not obtained from the same amount—i.e. if she had three beers daily, at one point, three beers wouldn't work anymore because she became tolerant to it, and she would have to drink four or five to get the same effect.

Withdrawal refers to the physical withdrawal that people can go through if they do not have enough of a drug that they are dependent on—i.e. if she drank five beers daily, and then stopped, she could go into alcohol withdrawal, and get shaky, agitated and irritable. When you consider someone to be "addicted," that is called substance dependence.

When ADD is present with substance abuse or dependence, there are several aspects to consider when treating both.

The first question is: are ADD and the substance abuse/dependence related?

The answer is yes. I regularly see teens in my office who have ADD, and get high on marijuana daily. When I ask them why they smoke "weed," they don't say: "It's because I want to sit around and giggle with my friends," they say: "because it relaxes me." They are using the drugs to self medicate their hyperactivity and agitation. Teens will often try to convince me that marijuana improves their focus as well. I explain that the research is quite clear that marijuana lowers their thinking abilities and memory, but it may feel like they can concentrate, because they are less hyperactive and restless.

Newer research has shown that when we treat ADD effectively, we can lower the risk of ADD kids developing drug and alcohol problems in adolescence and adult life. Please consider this as a benefit of medication treatment for ADD, particularly if you have a family history of drug and alcohol problems. Years ago, parents were reluctant to give their kids Ritalin®, because they thought their kids would become addicted to it. If medications are taken as prescribed, they do not cause a "high" and they are not habit forming. Long term studies show that when kids take the old medications like Ritalin®, they significantly decrease the risk of drug and alcohol problems later in adolescence. This data helps to confirm the fact that when we treat ADD effectively, we reduce the risk of drug and alcohol problems.

If ADD and substance abuse/dependence are present together, the doctor will have to decide which needs treatment first. This will relate to which condition is causing the most difficulties, or which one will result in the better outcome more readily. To a large extent, this depends on the substance abused, and the severity of the substance abuse or dependence.

If someone is addicted to heroin, cocaine or crystal meth, then they need *immediate* medical care and addiction treatment. ADD is something to be handled when they are more stable, and not actively using drugs.

If someone is smoking marijuana daily, then their ADD can be treated. Contrary to what parents want me to tell their teens—in general, the use of ADD medications and marijuana will not seriously harm their teen—i.e. it doesn't cause brain damage, or liver problems or anything like that. I explain to teens that the marijuana is not helping them, and, in fact, it undermines the medicine's effect. I encourage teens to reduce or stop their marijuana use. Please check with your doctor for specific advice for your child or teen.

Research in substance dependence with teens shows that a "harm reduction" treatment model is often better than an "abstinence" treatment model. If the treatment approach says that the teen has to immediately stop all use of the marijuana (or any other drug for that matter), then the teen is less likely to comply and succeed (the abstinence model). Compare this to an approach which educates the teen and gives him strategies to use less of the drug, while setting targets to aim for. This is the harm reduction model. In teens who use marijuana daily, the first step may be to not smoke it in the morning, and then not during school hours. The next goal may be to avoid smoking marijuana at all on weekdays, and so on.

If there is active alcohol use, it may be important to stop the alcohol use before treating the ADD. There are different patterns of alcohol dependence—daily use, vs. binge drinking. Binge drinking refers to people who abuse too much alcohol in binges—i.e. on the weekends. Depending on the circumstances, your doctor may recommend alcohol treatment first, or ADD treatment first. As a general rule of thumb, if the alcohol use is severe and problematic, then it will have to be dealt with first. If it is more mild, then the ADD can be dealt with first.

There are many drugs like ecstasy (often called "E," or "X"), LSD (often called "acid"), and Ketamine (often called "special K") which are used on weekends for parties by teens who abuse drugs. If your teen is using these, the doctor will have to review the risks and benefits of using ADD medications. Generally speaking, the doctor will consider using ADD medicines if there is not very regular or daily use of these drugs.

One important point about using ADD medications when a teen is abusing drugs or alcohol: it is important for the teen to understand that the "high" that they get may be different, or they may get more side effects from their drug of abuse when they are on ADD medications. In other words, they may get high more quickly, or they may get more nauseous, etc.

Although medically it is ideal to not be taking any psychoactive drugs when taking ADD medications, the reality is that if teens think that they can't use any drugs at all while taking ADD medications, they will stop their medications so that they can continue to use drugs with their friends when they want to. After realizing this in my first year of practice, I reviewed the literature, and came forth with the opinion that I have described above.

Takeaways from Step 7: Treatment Integration

Finding the "best" treatment for ADD can be a constant challenge, due to the fact that so many things can change over time. It can feel like the finish line is moving, because, once things get stable for a while, things change again and then the stability may not be there. It is important to be aware of the need for treatment integration based on the different treatment options available, and what happens over time.

The factors we've reviewed which can impact treatment integration over time include:

1. The decisions you make, and the approaches you take
2. The resources available in your community
3. Growth and development of your child over time

4. Social and family factors

5. School factors

6. The co-existing conditions which may be present now, or which may come in the future

This is why treatment for ADD requires vigilance, and close monitoring over time. It is so important for parents to actively participate in the "Parent's ADD Journey," of going from *student* to *expert* to *advocate*, and to continually learn. This is one of the main factors which will help you to ensure your child's success over the years.

CHAPTER 10

Is ADD a Gift?

a s I have in this book, repeatedly explained to you, ADD is a real medical condition which can cause significant difficulties if it is not treated effectively. It is a brain-based condition, it is genetically passed down in families and it responds to proven treatments (like therapy, medications, and even alternatives).

Despite the fact that ADD is a real medical disorder, there are authors who have written about ADD as a gift. Why would they do this?

Any medical condition can cause significant challenges for the person diagnosed with it—including pain, decreased functioning, or even death. When it comes to diseases like cancer, heart disease or arthritis, it is hard to say that these conditions have a "gift" in them. They clearly cause pain and suffering and potentially even loss of life.

When it comes to a disorder like ADD, which affects people's thinking, feeling and personality, there may actually be a gift wrapped inside of it. This relates to the fact that people with ADD can see the world in a different way. They can see things from "outside the box," and that different approach can lead to dramatic changes in how we approach challenges and issues in our world.

There are a number of people online who speculate about whether famous historical figures had ADD. Of course there is no way to know, but when we read these people's stories, we can see that many of the people who made dramatic differences in our society (and history) seem like they had ADD.

Thomas Edison is an example of one such historical figure. He was a man who lived from 1847 to 1931. He was an inventor, scientist and businessman who is credited with inventing the phonograph, the motion picture camera and the light bulb amongst many other inventions which have changed lives around the globe.

Edison only stayed in school for three months, during which his teacher said he had trouble focusing. His mother took him home and homeschooled him. He explored his interests and developed his own way of learning. Many experts who have read his early story suggest he likely would have been diagnosed with ADD based on the symptoms described.

As one who thought differently than others of his time, Edison developed ideas, technologies and inventions which propelled our world forward in dramatic ways. He founded the large company General Electric. He was a very successful and influential man. He was described as someone who thought differently than other people, and this was likely due to his unique brain—which was possibly due to ADD.

Others—contemporary, well known people—have come forward to share the fact that they themselves have ADD. Michael Phelps, the American Olympic swimmer who won eight gold medals in Beijing has ADD. Howie Mandel, the actor and comedian, has come forward and shared he has ADD. And so has *Extreme Makeover: Home Edition* host, Ty Pennington.

These celebrities coming forward and sharing that they have ADD is important for a number of reasons. Firstly, it helps to destigmatize ADD. Secondly, it shows young people what is possible when you have ADD. One could argue that Edison's creative problem solving, Phelp's complete dedication to his sport (hyperfocus), Mandel's quick creative humor (impulsivity gone right) and Pennington's tremendous energy when rebuilding a house in just a few days (hyperactivity) relates directly to their ADD.

ADD may have a gift wrapped inside of it.

The challenge is that it is wrapped with a real medical condition which can cause serious consequences if it isn't treated properly.

You may be wondering how ADD symptoms could even be considered a gift. Let's look at the three main ADD symptoms: **inattention**, **hyperactivity** and **impulsivity**.

Inattention often comes out as kids and teens having trouble paying attention in class. What if they aren't focusing in class because they are thinking about the point being discussed from multiple angles? (Has your ADD child ever asked you more questions than you have patience for on a particular topic?) Or they are thinking of all of the different things that this one idea may relate to—i.e. rather than sticking to the one issue that the teacher wants them to, they are brainstorming all of the other things that this may relate to in a seemingly "distracted" way.

How can this be a gift? Inattention can be out-of-the-box thinking, problem solving differently, and relating things in different ways than others did (as Edison did, to invent so many incredible technologies). These traits can often be tremendously valued in a business or "real world" environment; however, they can be seriously problematic in a standard school environment.

Hyperactivity often demonstrates itself with kids being restless and not sitting still in class. What's the gift? Increased energy. This can be a great gift, but only if the energy is harnessed productively.

Impulsivity often comes out as kids interrupting, or acting before thinking. How can this be a gift? Creativity can be said to be impulsivity gone right. Also, an ADD individual *can* avoid getting caught in "paralysis of analysis," and make a choice and move forward. This is another trait which can be highly valued in a business or real life environment, though not necessarily valued in the schools.

Do these comments above prove that ADD is a gift?

Absolutely not! They describe how people with ADD can look to harness the unique nature of their minds to benefit from their ADD traits. This does not mean that ADD is a gift. It only means that it *can* be.

As mentioned previously, ADD can have gifts inside of it, though they can be hard to unwrap. There are six steps one can use to unwrap the gifts of ADD.

The first step to unwrapping the gifts of ADD is to recognize that to make ADD a gift, one has to work hard at keeping the symptoms out of the way. If one is so symptomatic that he's having trouble functioning day-to-day, even if he has the gift of creativity, he can't harness it due to the symptoms interfering. Therefore the first step to unwrapping the gift of ADD is to treat the symptoms so that they are only traits. This is not only the first step, but it is actually necessary to even find the gifts in ADD. If one is dealing with the consequences of the disorder of ADD regularly, there is no way to even see the gift that can be inside of ADD.

The second step to unwrapping the gifts in ADD is to have the right supports around your son or daughter. The right supports will help your child to succeed, and to increase the chances of maintaining success from day-to-day as he or she progresses in life. The right supports also help to keep the symptoms at bay so that they don't interfere. By following the seven steps in the Attention Difference Disorder System, you'll know the right supports which need to be there.

The third step to unwrapping the gifts in ADD is to find your child's strengths and passions. You need to actively pursue different areas until your child finds something they love. It could be football, karate lessons, playing the piano, writing, art, chess or even debating. It doesn't matter what it is. You need to actively pursue it with your child until you find it. I have had many parents in my office telling me about all of the different lessons and activities they have tried with their child without success. My message to them is simple: keep trying. When your child finds something that she's truly passionate about it, she can concentrate on it easily, enjoy it readily, and want to progress through the challenging parts and develop skill. This is so important, because when one grows through further learning, that is how self esteem develops.

The fourth step to unwrapping the gifts in ADD is to develop and maximize the passions that your child has found in Step 3. Find lessons for him. Find a mentor who can guide him. Get books, or supplies or DVDs which teach him more. This will build his passion, skill, enjoyment and self esteem. Although it would be great if your child were great at and loved many things, all that is needed is one (and playing video games for hours doesn't count!). You need to nurture it and support it.

The fifth step is to embrace your child's ADD traits and celebrate his differences. By this I mean for you to change your child's perspective of it. This will help to destigmatize it. Make ADD something that is notable, worthy and supported, rather than a negative disorder which is ruining his life. This shift in perspective can make a dramatic difference in his life over the years. Realize that this has to be done after at least, the negative symptoms are treated.

Once the negative symptoms are treated, then it is easier to change the perspective about ADD. While someone is completely symptomatic of ADD and "suffering" the consequences of the symptoms, it is unrealistic to say that ADD is a great and wonderful gift. That idea is frankly insulting to your child's intelligence. Once you can control the symptoms (Step 1), get the right supports (Step 2), find the passions (Step 3) and nurture the passions (Step 4), then it can make sense to see the possible gifts in ADD—by pointing out how your child's unique thinking contributes to the great things he or she is accomplishing.

The sixth and final step is to continually revisit this—i.e. repeat Steps 1 through 5. As we reviewed in Step 7 of the Attention Difference Disorder System, Treatment Integration, you need to monitor and adjust treatment for ADD over time. To unwrap the gifts of ADD, you'll need to revisit Steps 1 through 5 over and over again.

The six steps to unwrap the gifts of ADD are summarized here:

1. Get the negative symptoms out of the way—turn the "disorder" into "traits."

2. Have the right supports around your child or teen.

3. Find your child's strengths and passions.

4. Develop and maximize these passions.

5. Embrace your child's ADD—celebrate his or her differences.

6. Keep revisiting Steps 1 through 5.

Is There Scientific Proof that ADD is a Gift?

While I have seen a few studies which tried to examine the creativity or problem solving abilities of people with ADD, they were not impressive, and it was hard to draw firm conclusions from these studies.

The short answer is this: there is no scientific proof that ADD is a gift. There is no proof that it provides any advantage to those who have it.

Critics of this chapter will no doubt challenge me as a physician discussing an unproven idea that ADD is a gift. They will say that I am actually undermining the nature of the disorder and setting it backwards. When this happens, I will listen politely, and continue to share this message—that ADD *can* be a gift.

Medical colleagues may challenge this idea as well. In medicine, there is a concept called the "standard of care." If someone has a medical mishap, the medical board (or the courts) will review if the doctor has met the "standard of care" with that patient. While there are more complex explanations, the standard of care at its core is: what would 100 other doctors in the same field do (or believe)? I know that most of the doctors in the field of ADD do not consider ADD a gift. They consider it a disorder which needs treatment, and they would most likely mock the idea that ADD is a gift. And yet, if they do, I will listen politely, and continue to share this message—that ADD *can* be a gift.

Why do I hold onto the belief that ADD can be a gift, despite the external pressures which would encourage me to stop thinking this way?

It is directly related to my experiences with hundreds of young people with ADD. When I see kids and teens who overcome their symptoms, and go on to achieve incredible things, they inspire me. After talking to lots of them—about what worked for them, and how they got from symptomatic to successful—I developed this perspective. If they could get the main treatment in place (i.e. the seven steps of the Attention Difference Disorder System) and then take the view that ADD can be a gift (the six steps to unwrapping the gifts of ADD), then they began to succeed. Their unique talents came out, they persisted with their goals, and they achieved more than they could have imagined.

One of my biggest concerns with ADD is when the young person experiences shame and guilt around their ADD. These thinking patterns with ADD can completely undermine a young person's potential—both in the present and in the future. It can take a lot of work to unwrap the gifts of ADD, but it is worth it.

So … I persist with the message: ADD *can* be a gift, but it can take a lot of work.

Maybe ADD Isn't a Gift: You Decide

To help you to decide if you want to consider ADD a gift, let's do a classic logic experiment. It's a 2 x 2 grid which looks at whether ADD is a gift or not, and whether you believe it is. In this experiment, there are four possibilities:

1. You believe ADD is a gift, and it is.
2. You believe ADD is a gift, and it isn't.
3. You don't believe ADD is a gift, and it is.
4. You don't believe ADD is a gift, and it isn't.

In possibility #1, you believe that ADD is a gift and it is. In this circumstance, you are now providing support and encouragement in a way which inspires your son or daughter, and helps to give them opportunities and options that they didn't even realize. You are happy that you considered ADD a gift, because it has paid off.

In possibility #2, you believe that ADD is a gift and it isn't. In this circumstance, you have provided encouragement, support and a non-stigmatizing approach to ADD for your child or teen. ADD really isn't a gift, so some of your enthusiasm is wasted, and your child may have considered you terribly embarrassing and annoying at times. In this situation, you risk putting too much energy into something that isn't right (i.e. considering ADD a gift).

In possibility #3, you believe that ADD is a not a gift, and it is. In this circumstance, you are not putting any energy or thought into ADD being a gift. You view all of the negatives of the condition, and you repeat these regularly to anyone who will listen. You work hard to get treatment for your son or daughter, and your child knows that they have a terrible disorder with awful consequences called ADD. In this circumstance of the logic experiment, ADD is actually a gift. This would lead to many missed possibilities and opportunities. There may even be consequences to this—i.e. your child may not go as far as they could have, because of their belief in the limitations of their ADD.

In possibility #4, you believe that ADD is not a gift, and it isn't. In this circumstance, you have saved yourself any wasted energy and time on an idea which was wrong. You didn't get "too positive" and you didn't push your child to pursue any passions of theirs unnecessarily. You can feel good about the fact that you were right—ADD is all negative.

Based on this logic experiment above, you can *choose* whether you want to consider ADD a gift, and whether you want to follow the steps to unwrapping the gifts of ADD. It is my personal opinion and choice that I consider that ADD can be a gift, and I encourage others to do so as well. I tend to be an optimist, and I work hard to help others to find the positive aspects of their challenges. That is one of the traits that I consider crucial in my profession as a psychiatrist. (Who wants to see a psychiatrist who is a pessimist and only focuses on the negative? Especially if he or she is working with kids...)

The ultimate answer is: there is no proof that ADD is a gift. Considering ADD as a gift is a choice. A choice that I encourage you to make to improve your child's life over the long term. There is little to lose, and potentially a lot to gain.

CHAPTER 11

What to Do Now?

C ongratulations on finishing this book. As the parent of a child or teen with ADD, your time is precious, and I commend you on finishing this book.

Right now, you know a lot more than many doctors about ADD. You now know more than many teachers. And you certainly know more about ADD than most of your family members.

What do you need to do now?

You need to start to implement what you've learned. In fact, I hope you haven't waited until the end of the book to start to use the information that you've learned to help your son or daughter.

Remember that there are no perfect treatment plans or approaches. Start implementing the strategies you've learned to the best of your ability, and monitor how they are helping. If they are working, keep going. If they aren't, then just re-evaluate them.

Be sure to get help from the professionals in your community, like the doctors, psychologists, behavioral therapists, educators, tutors, ADD coaches, etc. Remember to find a parent support group. If you can find one locally, it can help you tremendously. If you can't find a local one, use the power of the Internet to find some parents to share with and to support one another on your journey of helping your son or daughter with ADD. The Internet isn't just a window; it is a door to the world dealing with your concerns.

Remember to actively follow and embrace the ADD Parent's Journey of going from *student* to *expert* to *advocate*. This is a journey that I am personally on each day. I am a constant student (continually reading more about ADD, learning from the families that I work with, and attending conferences); I am an expert and an advocate as well. I hope you join me on this path.

How do you advocate effectively? Start by helping your son or daughter get what they need in your community. This is very important advocacy work! As you begin to succeed with that, then consider sharing with other parents how they can use similar strategies to help their kids. Consider sharing the ideas that you've learned from this book to teach people what they need to know about ADD. This helps to destigmatize ADD, and it is only by enough people standing up and breaking down misinformation that we can really destigmatize this condition. This improves things for your own child, as well as many other kids, teens and adults with ADD.

Finally, I encourage you to remember that there can be differences rather than deficits, and you need to maintain a strength-based approach to ADD. You can choose to see the positive aspects of ADD once you treat it effectively, and you can choose to consider it a gift. And by following the seven simple steps in the Attention Difference Disorder System, you can make a tremendous difference in your child or teen's life.

About the Author

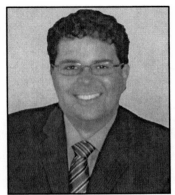

d
r. Kenny Handelman, a Child, Adolescent and Adult Psychiatrist, is an expert in ADHD —board certified in the USA and Canada. He is an Adjunct Professor of Psychiatry at the University of Western Ontario. He teaches other doctors, residents and medical students, as well as parents, educators and kids/teens about ADHD. He speaks internationally about ADHD, and does clinical research in the subject. He is often interviewed for TV and Radio about ADHD. He writes a widely read ADHD blog, getting over 500,000 visitors per year. Dr. Handelman's strength-based approach to ADHD is well received by parents of kids and teens, as it provides a practical approach which includes specifics on how to achieve success.

Index

Bonus: Free Audio Training for Parents

"Make a Difference in 7 Steps"
CLAIM YOUR FREE AUDIO TRAINING
on How to Make A Difference In Your Child's Life

As you read this book, you'll get the important tools and strategies to help your child or teen with ADD/ADHD.

You'll also get the right *perspective* on how to view ADD - to move from a deficit model to a differences model. You'll learn how to turn your child's deficits into differences, and his / her differences into strengths.

In this free bonus audio training, I'll help you to take the learning from this book "off the page" and into your child or teen's life. And that's what you really need - strategies that you can act on, which change your child or teen's life (and your family's life) for the better.

Claim Your Free Audio Training Today:

www.AttentionDifferenceDisorder.com/Bonus

Extra Bonus:

Claim Your FREE Membership To The Attention Difference Disorder® Online Community

Our online community will allow you to join other like minded people who take action to improve life for people with ADD.

BUY A SHARE OF THE FUTURE IN YOUR COMMUNITY

These certificates make great holiday, graduation and birthday gifts that can be personalized with the recipient's name. The cost of one S.H.A.R.E. or one square foot is $54.17. The personalized certificate is suitable for framing and

will state the number of shares purchased and the amount of each share, as well as the recipient's name. The home that you participate in "building" will last for many years and will continue to grow in value.

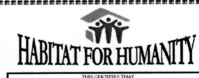

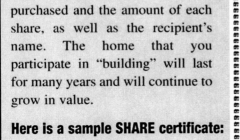

THIS CERTIFIES THAT

YOUR NAME HERE

HAS INVESTED IN A HOME FOR A DESERVING FAMILY

1985-2005

TWENTY YEARS OF BUILDING FUTURES IN OUR COMMUNITY ONE HOME AT A TIME

1200 SQUARE FOOT HOUSE @ $65,000 = $54.17 PER SQUARE FOOT
This certificate represents a tax deductible donation. It has no cash value.

Here is a sample SHARE certificate:

YES, I WOULD LIKE TO HELP!

I support the work that Habitat for Humanity does and I want to be part of the excitement! As a donor, I will receive periodic updates on your construction activities but, more importantly, I know my gift will help a family in our community realize the dream of homeownership. **I would like to SHARE in your efforts against substandard housing in my community!** *(Please print below)*

PLEASE SEND ME _____ SHARES at $54.17 EACH = $ $_____

In Honor Of: _____

Occasion: (Circle One)   HOLIDAY   BIRTHDAY   ANNIVERSARY

    OTHER: _____

Address of Recipient: _____

Gift From: _____ *Donor Address:* _____

Donor Email: _____

I AM ENCLOSING A CHECK FOR $ $_____ PAYABLE TO HABITAT FOR HUMANITY <u>OR</u> PLEASE CHARGE MY VISA OR MASTERCARD *(CIRCLE ONE)*

Card Number _____ Expiration Date: _____

Name as it appears on Credit Card _____ Charge Amount $ _____

Signature _____

Billing Address _____

Telephone # Day _____ Eve _____

PLEASE NOTE: Your contribution is tax-deductible to the fullest extent allowed by law.
Habitat for Humanity • P.O. Box 1443 • Newport News, VA 23601 • 757-596-5553
www.HelpHabitatforHumanity.org

CPSIA information can be obtained at www.ICGtesting.com
Printed in the USA
BVOW041033070213

312666BV00001B/153/P

9 781600 378881